"Impressive. In

—ROBER̲... ...I OM AC Kt FRS. President of the Royal Society, ... Chief Scientific Advisor to the UK government (1995–2000). Lord May is currently at the forefront of global warming research and is considered a pioneer in epidemiological research.

"Dr. Pierpont has clinically defined a new group of human subjects who respond to low frequency, relatively high amplitude forces acting upon the sensory and other body systems. Her rigorous clinical observations are consistent with reports of the deleterious effects of infrasound on humans, including, but not limited to, the low frequency sonar effects on divers. There are clinical conditions (such as dehiscent superior semicircular canals) that might explain some of Dr. Pierpont's clinical symptom review, but this relatively rare condition cannot explain all of her observations.

"Dr. Pierpont's astute collection of observations should motivate a well-controlled, multi-site, multi-institutional prospective study."

—F. OWEN BLACK, MD, FACS, Senior Scientist and Director of Neuro-Otology Research, Legacy Health System, Portland, Oregon. Dr. Black is widely considered to be one of the foremost balance, spatial orientation, and equilibrium clinical researchers in America.

"Like so many earlier medical pioneers exposing the weaknesses of current orthodoxy, Dr. Nina Pierpont has been subjected to much denigration and criticism. It is a tribute to her strength of character and conviction that this important book has reached publication. Her detailed recording of the harm caused by wind turbine noise will lay firm foundations for future research. It should be required reading for all planners considering 'wind farms.'"

—CHRISTOPHER HANNING, MD, FRCA, MRCS, LRCP. Dr. Hanning, a founder of the British Sleep Society, is a leading sleep clinician and researcher. He recently retired as Director of the Sleep Clinic and Laboratory at Leicester General Hospital, one of the largest sleep disorder clinics in the UK.

"This is an extraordinary book. It is personal and passionate, which makes it compelling reading. But it is much more—authoritative, meticulous, and scholarly. The descriptions of anatomy, physiology, and the pathophysiology of how noise affects health are bang on. It clearly takes its place as the leading work on the topic.

"In addition to Dr. Pierpont's detailed clinical accounts, there is accumulating evidence of adverse health effects from Japan, New Zealand, the UK, USA, and Canada. There are also some 357 organizations from 19 European countries demanding an enquiry by the European Union about health and many other adverse effects of wind farms. At a minimum, the EU would be wise to consult with Dr. Pierpont.

"This book is a must-read for all health care professionals, especially those in clinical practice. One cannot but hope that politicians and policy makers at all levels heed the wake-up call that there are serious consequences to precipitant decisions relating to so-called green energy."

—ROBERT Y. McMURTRY, MD, FRCS (C), FACS. Former Dean of Medicine and Dentistry at the Schulich School of Medicine & Dentistry, University of Western Ontario. Dr. McMurtry has had a long and distinguished career in Canadian public health policy at both the federal and provincial level, including as founding Assistant Deputy Minister of the Population and Public Health Branch of Health Canada, and currently as a member of the Health Council of Canada.

"Dr. Pierpont has written a superb and powerful book. Truly first-rate in its presentation of hard data, and with remarkable clarity.

"I devoutly hope that her findings, pinned as they are to unassailable research and rigorously peer-reviewed by ranking scientists, come to the attention of movers and shakers who can broaden the research base and shape the politics of dealing with Wind Turbine Syndrome."

—JACK G. GOELLNER, Director Emeritus, The Johns Hopkins University Press (America's oldest university press, founded 1878). During Mr. Goellner's tenure as director, JHUP became a world leader, celebrated for its medical publishing, among other fields.

"Dr. Pierpont has made an important contribution to a debate about wind turbines that should be conducted not between champions and opponents of renewable energy, but within the community of those who want this country to behave in an environmentally responsible way. That we can and should do."

—EDITORIAL BOARD OF THE INDEPENDENT (UK), August 2, 2009

NINA PIERPONT, MD, PHD

Wind Turbine Syndrome

A Report on a Natural Experiment

K-Selected Books
Santa Fe, NM

Copyright © 2009 by Nina Pierpont.
All rights reserved.
This book may not be reproduced, in whole or in part, including illustrations, in any form (beyond that copying permitted by Sections 107 and 108 of the U.S. Copyright Law and except by reviewers for the public press), without written permission from the publishers. This prohibition specifically extends to Google Book Search and any other book search services.

Designed and set in Warnock type by Jordan Klassen.
Printed in the United States of America by King Printing, Lowell, Mass.

Publisher's Cataloging-in-Publication Data
(Provided by Quality Books, Inc.)

Pierpont, Nina.
    Wind turbine syndrome : a report on a natural experiment / Nina Pierpont.
       p. cm.
    Includes bibliographical references.
    ISBN-13: 978-0-9841827-0-1
    ISBN-10: 0-9841827-0-5

    1. Vestibular apparatus—Diseases. 2. Wind turbines—Health aspects. 3. Syndromes. I. Title.

RF260.P54 2009   617.8'82
                          QBI09-600120

10 9 8 7 6 5 4 3 2 1

This study is dedicated to the memory of Dudley Weider, MD, Professor of Otolaryngology at the Dartmouth-Hitchcock Medical Center, who sent me to Alaska, diagnosed and cured my husband, and taught me about migraine and dizziness. We miss him.

Contents

One	By way of explaining why on earth I wrote this book	1
Two	The Report, for clinicians	26
Three	The Case Histories: The raw data	126
Four	The Report all over again, in plain English for non-clinicians	193
Abbreviations		257
Glossary		259
References		271
Referee reports		287
About the author		293

ONE

By way of explaining why on earth I wrote this book

I wrote this report because I saw a medical problem that few clinicians were paying attention to or, for that matter, seemed to understand. Dr. Amanda Harry in the United Kingdom led the way in recognizing the cluster of symptoms people experience around wind turbines.[1] I, myself, began encountering the problem from numerous emails and telephone calls I began receiving in 2004, shortly after wind developers turned up in my community and my husband and I started investigating industrial wind turbines.

The uniformity of the complaints quickly became apparent. It didn't take long to realize the potential for a relationship between these complaints, on the one hand, and *migraine, motion sickness, vertigo, noise and visual and gastrointestinal sensitivity,* and *anxiety,* which, taken together, form a coherent and interconnected neurologic complex in medical practice.

The breakthrough came in early 2006, when I interviewed a couple who were about to move out of their home because of their own and their children's symptoms. The interview supported the

---

[1] Harry, Amanda. 2007. Wind turbines, noise, and health. 32 pp. www.windturbinenoisehealthhumanrights.com/wtnoise_health_2007_a_barry.pdf.

relationship between turbine-associated symptoms and migraine/motion sensitivity. Best of all, the interview introduced me to the curious phenomenon of vibration or pulsation felt in the chest. It was this element that caught the attention of the National Academy of Sciences in its 2007 report to Congress, *Environmental Impacts of Wind-Energy Projects*. The authors wanted to learn more about this effect of low frequency noise.[2]

This study is my answer to their question.

As I have worked to understand these complaints, I have benefited from new research allowing us to better understand neurologic phenomena like spatial memory loss and fear reactions in people with balance problems—symptoms that often "bored and baffled" clinicians, as one of my referees put it.[3] Wind developers and acousticians have been even less charitable:

> It's ... worth noting that studies have shown that a person's attitude toward a sound—meaning whether it's a "wanted" or "unwanted" sound—depends a great deal on what they think and how they feel about the source of the sound. In other words, if someone has a negative attitude to wind turbines, or is worried about them, this will affect how they feel about the sound. However, if someone has

---

[2] National Research Council. 2007. *Environmental Impacts of Wind-Energy Projects.* The National Academies Press, Washington, DC. 185 pp, p. 109 (Prepublication Copy). "Low-frequency vibration and its effects on humans are not well understood. Sensitivity to such vibration resulting from wind-turbine noise is highly variable among humans. Although there are opposing views on the subject, it has recently been stated (Pierpont 2006) that 'some people feel disturbing amounts of vibration or pulsation from wind turbines, and can count in their bodies, especially their chests, the beats of the blades passing the towers, even when they can't hear or see them.' More needs to be understood regarding the effects of low-frequency noise on humans" (pp. 108–9).

[3] I review and discuss this research in the Discussion section, p. 70.

a positive attitude toward wind energy, it's very unlikely that the sounds will bother them at all.[4]

Their patients [people living near wind turbines and reported on by Drs. Osborne and Harry] may well have been experiencing adverse symptoms, but we have to keep in mind that people who have failed, for whatever reason, in strong objections to a development, build up in themselves a level of unfulfilled expectations and consequent stress, which peaks after the failure and can overload their coping capabilities. This leads them to lay the blame on whatever straw they can clutch. This is especially so in group activities, where mutual support may turn to a mutual, interacting misery, which worsens the situation.... The very low levels of low frequency noise and infrasound which occur from wind turbines will not normally cause problems. If problems have occurred, it is possibly for some other stress-related reason.[5]

Brian Howe, a consulting engineer in acoustics for 20 years for HGC Engineering, said Ontario's guidelines for turbine noise are adequate and consistent with Health Canada studies. Most people near wind turbines aren't complaining about the noise, Howe said. In some cases, noise complaints could reflect higher anxiety levels from people who had unrealistic expectations of hearing virtually no sound, he said.[6]

---

[4] Noble Environmental Power, LLC. Wind fact sheet #5: Are modern wind turbines noisy? p. 2. www.windturbinesyndrome.com/?p=698.

[5] Leventhall, Geoff. 2004. Notes on low frequency noise from wind turbines with special reference to the Genesis Power Ltd. Proposal near Waiuku, NZ. Prepared for Genesis Power/Hegley Acoustic Consultants, June 4, p. 7.

[6] Rennie, Gary. 2009. Wind farm noise limits urged. *The Windsor Star* (Ontario, Canada). February 24.

Responses like these are a pity. They're rubbish. There is nothing "psychosomatic" or malingering about it. The physiologic pathway flows from physical forces (air pressure changes, noise, vibration) to physical sensations (chest pulsations, internal vibration, tinnitus, headache, ear fullness) to brain integration of sensory signals to distortions of brain functioning (sleeplessness, concentration and memory deficits, physical symptoms of anxiety)—not the reverse. Research clearly shows there are precise and definable neurologic connections that explain how distorted sensory signals can derail normal psychological and cognitive function and, in fact, trigger physical symptoms. (It's worth pointing out that our understanding of brain function has progressed by leaps and bounds in the last 25 years, radically changing the landscape of psychology and psychiatry and, of course, neurology.[7] Much of the research on vestibular function, whereon I draw, is even more recent, conducted within just the last 10–15 years.)

Leaving the pop psychology behind us, let's move on to evidence-based science. In the world of medicine my study is properly called a "case series," defined as *a descriptive account of a series of individuals with the same new medical problem*. Let me be clear: a case series is a standard and valid form of medical research. New illnesses are often introduced with case series whose role is to define an illness, suggest causation, and alert the medical and research profession to its existence. (This being one of the chief reasons for this report.) After an illness is defined and awareness raised, it becomes more feasible to do larger, more expensive studies to explore etiology (causation), pathophysiology, and epidemiologic characteristics.

---

[7] See, for example, Schore, Allan N. 1994. *Affect Regulation and the Origin of the Self: The Neurobiology of Emotional Development*. Lawrence Earlbaum Associates, Hillsdale, NJ. 700 pp.

Case series don't typically have control groups. Nevertheless, I saw I needed a comparison group of similar, though unexposed, people to distinguish which symptoms were due to turbine exposure. The most similar unexposed people, of course, were my study subjects themselves prior to turbine exposure and after the end of exposure. I therefore set up a *before-during-after* study format, interviewing families who had already moved out of their homes due to symptoms or who were planning to move and had already spent periods away from home, during which turbine-associated symptoms abated.

This format served a three-fold purpose:

1) it ensured there was an "after" phase for each family,
2) it guaranteed that at least one member of each family was severely affected, enough to need to move, and
3) it provided validation for participant statements, since one can hardly discount the gravity of symptoms that force a family to vacate its home or perform expensive renovations aimed solely at noise exclusion.

Which brings us to what is known in science as a "natural experiment": *a circumstance wherein subjects are exposed to experimental conditions both inadvertently and ecologically (within their own homes and environments)*. Obviously, it would be unethical to expose people deliberately to potentially harmful interventions. Hence natural experiments, while less controlled, have an important role in clarifying the impacts of potentially toxic, man-made exposures.

The ecological dimension in the phrase *natural experiment* is worth emphasizing, since many elements of an exposure may not be reproducible in a laboratory, such as round-the-clock exposure,

exposure over months, or impacts on customary activities. For symptoms related to wind turbine sound there are also technical difficulties in reproducing in a laboratory the types of sound, air pressure variation, and vibration that my subjects' observations suggest are involved. Failure to provoke the same symptoms in a laboratory setting may tell us more about the limitations of the laboratory situation than about real-world effects.

To further create comparison groups, I collected information on all members in the ten families, not just the most affected. This widened the age range of subjects and gave me information on variably affected people who were all exposed to turbine noise capable of causing severe symptoms. I then used the natural variation within the study group to examine which elements of the *pre-exposure* medical history predicted which parts of the *during-exposure* symptom complex. By this method the study begins to answer the intriguing question of why some individuals are affected more than others by living near wind turbines, and which individuals in the general population are notably at risk for symptoms. It also suggests pathophysiologic mechanisms.

It would be difficult to do a conventional epidemiologic study of the health effects of wind turbines, at least in the United States, even if one were blessed with substantial funding and institutional backing, as I was not. By "epidemiologic," I mean studies in which random or regular sampling is used (as, for example, assessing everyone within three miles of a set of turbines, or every fourth name in an alphabetical listing of everyone within three miles), or case and control populations identified. The difficulty comes from the legal and financial stone wall of the *gag clause*.

In the course of this study I repeatedly encountered these clauses in leases between wind developers and landowners, in "good neighbor" contracts between wind developers and neighbors to leaseholders, and in court decisions following citizen challenges to wind turbine development.[8] Gag clauses forbid people who receive payments from wind companies, or who have lost legal challenges, from saying anything negative about the turbines or developer.

Consider the following letter. It was written February 12, 2009, by a woman named Cheryl LeClair who lives in Altona, NY. Cheryl was in fact employed by the wind developer she was writing about, Noble Environmental Power, LLC, by whom she remained employed through January 2009. ("My employment ended on January 30th due to the end of the project and the economy. They [Noble] were a good employer" 2/12/09.) Her letter was not sent in confidence, being addressed as well to New York State Assemblywoman Janet Duprey and to Altona Town Supervisor Larry Ross, bearing the plea, "I am appealing for any help that you can give to me."

Cheryl begins by describing what life is like being surrounded by the turbines of the Noble Altona Wind Park.[9] "The visual effects of the windpark are very disorienting." The turbines "give me a feeling of motion sickness and dizziness. The sound on a breezy day like today is maddening. I have been told that I am in a unique position in which the sound reverberates/echoes/concentrates on my home. I am constantly expecting to see an airplane overhead."

Cheryl wrote to me, Duprey, and Ross because she felt her pleas to Noble were being ignored. In an earlier letter (1/26/09, included

---

[8] The "good neighbor agreements" go by various creative names, circumlocutions, and euphemisms.

[9] "With its excellent wind resources, the town of Altona is ideally positioned to benefit from a state-wide initiative to get more energy from renewable sources. Noble Environmental Power has built a 97.5 megawatt (MW) windpark using 65 GE 1.5 MW turbines.... On June 17, 2008, Noble held a groundbreaking ceremony to officially mark the start of construction" (www.noblepower.com).

with her 2/12/09 correspondence), she had informed Noble that "my head and body are trembling, dizzy, vibrating; the right way to describe what is happening to me right now eludes me. I do know that it is very uncomfortable.... This is unbearable." She compares her home to "an airport runway (lights), an airplane hovering overhead steadily, or an under-maintained amusement park ride (sounds), and a discotheque (flicker). I am emotionally and physically sick and distraught over this." Closing with, "I am at my wits end. I need solid answers from you, not [Noble employee's name withheld] calling and quoting what is in the town laws, studies from other areas, statements in the DEIS [Draft Environmental Impact Statement] and FEIS [Final EIS], etc. I am a real person with a REAL problem. I am asking very seriously for solutions, not rhetoric and quotes. Again, I invite any and all to come experience this first hand" (emphasis hers). "I also think that any future development team should be aware of and see the ramifications before this happens to someone else."

The 1/26/09 letter had been preceded a week and a half earlier (1/14/09) with this one (included with her 2/12/09 correspondence to me), likewise to Noble. "I can hear the 'whoosh, whoosh, whoosh' of the turbines from within my house," a noise that's "not anything like the steady hum of a refrigerator. While it may be no louder than that, there is NO comparison" (emphasis hers). "The wind park," she declares, "has completely ruined the quality of my life in this home that I love."

In a subsequent email to me, she described how her right ear "has been ringing steadily for three or so months. It never changes, never goes away," adding, "when I wake around 2:30 or 3:00, I find it nearly impossible to go back to sleep."

Cheryl doesn't have a name for her cluster of symptoms. But I do. It was after hearing from numerous Cheryl LeClairs that I coined the phrase "Wind Turbine Syndrome." Unfortunately, I will never get to study Cheryl's symptoms beyond these tantalizing emails. In an update she explains why:

> Mr. Ross sent my papers (easements) to two separate lawyers. *They both replied that I had signed away my rights and really had no leg to stand on.* Ms. Duprey sent me a letter that said *she spoke to Noble representatives and was told that because I had signed an easement, there was nothing she could do to help me.* . . . [Noble] approached me with an agreement to fix the TV reception and *reiterate the signing away of my rights.* Conundrum? Is that how you would say (and spell) it?? [Emphasis mine.]

"Conundrum"—yes, that's the word, and yes, that's how you spell it. "I did sign a 'border easement' with Noble, and I was an employee. I get $1,000/year until operational, then I will get $2,000/year" (2/12/09 letter).

Border Easement = Good Neighbor Agreement = Gag Clause.

Gag clauses encompass matters of health. And this, dear reader, explains why Cheryl LeClair, suffering from textbook Wind Turbine Syndrome, is not available for clinical study (at least public study). (When I studied public health in medical school, they didn't warn us about gag clauses.)

The punchline being that in an epidemiologic study based on interviews or questionnaires, gag clauses can easily distort answers or skew participation, invalidating a random sample.

Besides the gag clause, some people informed me that they didn't want to talk about their problems because they hoped to sell their homes in order to flee the turbines next door. (No better way to kill a real estate deal than to leak the news that one's home is toxic.) There is also the matter of relationships and family ties within small, close-knit communities, where folks are often reluctant to reveal a problem because, let's say, the turbines on your cousin's land happen to be the source of it.

In this manner has the wind industry both shattered many rural communities and thwarted research like mine.

Despite what I see as the virtues of my approach, this study has clear limitations. One being that it was conducted entirely by clinical interview, over the telephone. On the one hand this had the benefit of allowing me to have an international group of subjects. On the other it limited the type of data I could collect. As a result, my ability to say that *a certain symptom during exposure is due to turbines* is confined to medical conditions which are diagnosable by medical history. (A medical history is *all the information a patient tells the doctor about his illness, his past health and experiences, and his habits.*)

As an aside, non-clinicians should realize that in medicine many conditions (ailments) are diagnosed mostly by medical history. This includes migraine and other headaches, tinnitus, and sleep disturbance. (Medical diagnosis is not all x-rays and MRI's and lab tests.) It stands to reason that your doctor can't tell objectively (by any sort of clinical test) if you have a headache, tinnitus, or sleep problem, and much of what your doc figures out about the causes of these symptoms will come from the other questions he asks you. This is the part I could credibly do by telephone.

My study subjects also told me about other kinds of problems which seemed to worsen during exposure, including asthma, pneumonia, pleurisy, stroke, and changes in coagulation or blood sugar. I did not include these in Wind Turbine Syndrome, since my method of study did not allow me to determine whether in fact wind turbines played a role in these conditions during exposure. These conditions would require other kinds of study over and above the clinical interview and case series. (I have included them in a separate section of the *Results* in the REPORT FOR CLINICIANS because I think they may need attention from the medical research community.)

This study also does not tell us how many people are affected within a certain distance of wind turbines. But it does offer a framework for what to pursue in such a study (meaning, the next phase: epidemiologic studies), such as what symptoms to study and what aspects of the exposure to measure.

Shifting, now, to the format of the book. I wrote the REPORT FOR CLINICIANS as a (long) scientific article, beginning with an *Abstract* or brief summary, followed by an *Introduction* to the problem and background information, a description of the *Methods* used (including study sample selection), a presentation of the *Results* (which are the data secured during the study and its analysis), and finally *Discussion* of the results with interpretation of their meaning in the context of current medical knowledge. Data are compiled in *Tables* (numbered 1A, 1B, 1C, 2, and 3) included within the *Results* section.

REFERENCES are footnoted in the text and listed together towards the end of the book. I added a GLOSSARY of medical and technical terms to make the book more intelligible to non-medical readers, and a list of ABBREVIATIONS.

The CASE HISTORIES (A1 through J4) present the raw narrative data—each individual subject's symptoms and statements—in table format, one person per table with separate columns for *before*, *during*, and *after* exposure, and separate rows for each organ or functional system (sleep, headache, cognition, balance/equilibrium, ears/hearing, etc.).

The Case Histories are gathered together at the end of the clinical text. They are the backbone of my report. I deeply appreciate my subjects' willingness to be included herein.

The book is intended for physicians and other professionals and individuals who wish to better understand the wind turbine–associated symptom complex. This posed a dilemma: writing in the specialized language of clinical medicine and science is very different from the language one uses for laymen. Yet my goal is to reach both audiences. I solved the problem by adding (at my editor's insistence) a more conversational, parallel text, which I christened Report for Non-Clinicians.

The result is a book with two, tandem texts. They say the same thing. One says it in the language of the clinician (Report for Clinicians), the other in the everyday language of—well—my editor (Report for Non-Clinicians).

The goal of Report for Clinicians is scientific precision, including frequent expressions of my degree of certainty or uncertainty. Since the physics and the physiology I invoke are complex and not widely known among clinicians, I explain them in this text. Here, likewise, I quote and summarize numerous scientific articles, and I use numbers and statistics (albeit the simplest type known).

Report for Non-Clinicians says it all over again, this time in English my mother-in-law would understand. To accomplish this, I had to sacrifice a degree of scientific precision, since *plain English* and *scientific precision* don't always mix. I freely acknowledge that the Report for Non-Clinicians might set some clinicians' teeth on edge, and for this I beg their indulgence.

A second disclaimer. Readers should understand that Wind Turbine Syndrome is not the same as Vibroacoustic Disease.[10] I say this because the two are often equated in the popular media. The proposed mechanisms are different, and the noise amplitudes are probably different as well.

Wind Turbine Syndrome, I propose, is mediated by the vestibular system—by disturbed sensory input to eyes, inner ears, and stretch and pressure receptors in a variety of body locations. These feed back neurologically onto a person's sense of position and motion in space, which is in turn connected in multiple ways to brain functions as disparate as spatial memory and anxiety. Several lines of evidence suggest that the amplitude (power or intensity) of low frequency noise and vibration needed to create these effects may be even lower than the auditory threshold at the same low frequencies. Re-stating this, it appears that even low frequency noise or vibration too weak to be heard can still stimulate the human vestibular system, opening the door for the symptoms I call Wind Turbine Syndrome. I am happy to report there is now direct experimental evidence of such vestibular sensitivity in normal humans.[11]

Vibroacoustic Disease, on the other hand, is hypothesized to be caused by direct tissue damage to a variety of organs, creating thickening of supporting structures and other pathological changes.[12] The suspected agent is high amplitude (high power or intensity) low frequency noise. Given my research protocol, described above, my study is of course unable to demonstrate whether wind turbine exposure causes the types of pathologies

---

[10] Castelo Branco NAA, Alves-Pereira M. 2004. Vibroacoustic disease. Noise Health 6(23): 3–20.

[11] Todd NPMc, Rosengren SM, Colebatch JG. 2008. Tuning and sensitivity of the human vestibular system to low-frequency vibration. Neurosci Lett 444: 36–41.

[12] Castelo Branco and Alves-Pereira 2004.

found in Vibroacoustic Disease, although there are similarities that may be worthy of further clinical investigation, especially with regard to asthma and lower respiratory infections.

Moving on, I have been asked if Wind Turbine Syndrome could be caused by magnetic or electric fields. I have no reason to think so. There has been extensive epidemiologic research since 1979 on magnetic fields and health, comparing people who live close to high power lines or work in electrical utilities or work in other industries where magnetic field exposure is likely to be high, to people who do not.[13] This substantial body of research has produced no good evidence that magnetic field exposure causes cancer in children or adults, cardiac or psychiatric disease, dementia, or multiple sclerosis.[14,15] After three decades of research, there is still no experimental evidence for a physiologic mechanism for any of the proposed effects of magnetic fields.[16]

This makes it difficult to do epidemiologic studies, since researchers don't know what exposure to measure, or what exposure period (e.g., last week or five years ago) might be relevant.[17] An association has been shown between higher magnetic field exposure in utility workers and amyotrophic lateral sclerosis (ALS), a neurodegenerative disease, but this is most likely due to more frequent electric shocks in these settings, not to the magnetic

---

[13] Ahlbom IC, Cardis E, Green A, Linet M, Savitz D, Swerdlow A; INCIRP (International Commission for Non-Ionizing Radiation Protection) Standing Committee on Epidemiology. 2001. Review of the epidemiologic literature on EMF and health. Environ Health Perspect 109 Suppl 6: 911–33.

[14] Ahlbom et al. 2001.

[15] Johansen C. 2004. Electromagnetic fields and health effects: epidemiologic studies of cancer, diseases of the central nervous system and arrhythmia-related heart disease. Scand J Work Environ Health 30 Suppl 1: 1–30.

[16] Ahlbom et al. 2001.

[17] Ahlbom et al. 2001.

fields.[18] Claims that voltage and frequency irregularities in household alternating currents (what some refer to as "dirty electricity") create a wide, non-specific swath of medical problems—from ADHD to rashes to diabetes to cancer—are completely unsubstantiated, and also have no plausible biologic mechanisms.[19]

A few words about peer review. Peer review is quite simple, contrary to the mystique it has acquired among wind developers (most of whom probably have a fanciful idea of what it is). Peer review *consists of sending a scholarly manuscript to experts in that particular field of knowledge, who are asked to judge whether it merits publication.* Simple as that. The identity of reviewers (also called "referees") can be either known to the author (with book manuscripts, authors are routinely asked by editors to submit a list of recommended referees) or kept confidential.

If the referees (usually consisting of two or three) manage to convince the editor that the manuscript is not worthy of publication, the editor contacts the author and rejects the manuscript. If, on the other hand, the referees feel the manuscript merits publication subject to certain revisions and perhaps additions, the editor will forward their reports to the author and ask for a response. "Are you willing to make these changes? Do you agree with these criticisms? If not, give me compelling reasons why not."

The author then revises the manuscript accordingly, except where she feels her referees are wrong—and manages to convince the

---

[18] Johansen 2004.
[19] I have asked Prof. Magda Havas, Environmental and Resource Studies, Trent University, Ontario, Canada, to remove references to Wind Turbine Syndrome from her PowerPoint presentation on hypothesized wind turbine health effects, because these references are inaccurate.

editor. Once the editor feels the author has addressed criticisms and suggestions adequately, he (she) proceeds with publication.

Lastly, referees do not have to agree with the author's arguments or conclusions. This is worth emphasizing. Their purpose is merely to certify that a) the manuscript conforms to conventional standards of scholarly or clinical research appropriate to the discipline, and, perhaps most important, b) the manuscript is a significant contribution to knowledge.

In the case of this book, a variety of scientists and physicians, all professors at medical schools or university departments of biology, read and commented on the manuscript and recommended it as an important contribution to knowledge and conforming to the canons of clinical and scientific research. Moreover, they did in fact suggest revisions, even substantial revisions and additions, all of which I made. Some gave me written reports to include in the book itself. See REFEREE REPORTS. Others offered to review the book after it was published.

That said, the litmus test of scientific validity is not peer review, which, after all, is not infallible, as the history of science amply demonstrates. Peer review is an important first step in judging scientific or scholarly merit. Still, the ultimate test is whether other scientists can follow the author's research protocol and get the same results, or if different lines of research point to the same conclusions.

That, of course, remains to be seen with this report.

I thank Dr. Joel Lehrer in particular for providing me with new information regarding vestibular function, contributions echoed by Drs. Owen Black and Abraham Shulman (all in otolaryngology/neurotology). I thank Professors Ralph Katz (epidemiology) and

Henry Horn (ecology) for discussion of scientific method and presentation. Dr. Jerome Haller (neurology) and Professor Robert May (theoretical ecology and epidemiology, past president of the Royal Society of London) read the manuscript and provided commentary to be included in the book, as did Dr. Lehrer and Professors Katz and Horn, for which I am most grateful. Barbara Frey (biomedical librarian) edited the manuscript, and discovered and sent me many essential—indeed critical—references. Christina Ransom and William McCall, librarians of the Champlain Valley Physician's Hospital in Plattsburgh, NY, and the FYI Hospital Library Circuit Rider Program, sent countless articles by PDF and delivered several books. I am grateful for all their work and good humor, and for their program, which gives rural doctors access to the full medical and scientific literature.[20]

I also thank the other readers who read and discussed the manuscript with me and advised on routes of publication: Professor Carey Balaban (neuroscience), Dr. Rolf Jacob (psychiatry/neurotology interface), Dr. John Modlin (pediatrics/infectious diseases), and Dr. Anne Gadomski (pediatrics/public health).

George Kamperman, INCE (Institute of Noise Control Engineering) Board Certified noise control engineer, and Rick James, INCE Full Member, edited the sections describing noise measurement and modeling. They also analyzed noise studies done at the homes of several affected families, while developing standards and protocols for the assessment and control of noise from industrial wind turbines. Kamperman and James presented their standards and rationale at the Noise-Con 2008 meeting of the Institute of Noise Control Engineering (USA) in July 2008, then expanded their paper with a detailed discussion of noise measurement protocols and a

---

[20] While I'm acknowledging debts, I wish to thank R. Forrest Martin for the fine (and witty) drawings decorating the REPORT FOR NON-CLINICIANS, and I thank Jordan Klassen for his eye and care in designing this book.

model wind turbine ordinance.[21] The expanded paper is posted on the Wind Turbine Syndrome website.[22]

Some are surprised that I chose to publish this study as a book rather than an article. My reason is purely practical: it's too long for a medical or scientific journal. The problem is the incompressible yet indispensable narrative data—people's accounts of their sensations, experiences, symptoms, and history. It would be impossible to present these accounts in a 3000- or 7000-word article, yet they are essential as evidence for qualitative changes around turbines.

For example, to support a summary statement like "The noise from wind turbines has a different and disturbing quality, even when it does not seem loud," I must present the descriptions given by multiple study participants. Likewise, to describe a symptom new to medicine, such as the feeling of internal vibration or pulsation, I again need the words of multiple participants. Because I could not do testing to examine thinking and memory abilities, for example, I need to recount the subjects' own evidence, consisting of their descriptions of things they used to do easily but now cannot do, or of loss and recovery in their children's school functioning.

Many of my reviewers suggested ways to split the study into shorter papers. A segment on migraine, one on tinnitus, and another on methodology, for example. However, I feel that keeping the entire study in one piece makes for a more powerful and intelligible document, allowing readers to appreciate the intertwined nature of individual symptoms and the way they fit with new neural models of vestibular function.

---

[21] Kamperman GW, James RR. 2008a. Simple guidelines for siting wind turbines to prevent health risks. Noise-Con, July 28–31, Institute of Noise Control Engineering/USA.

[22] See "How loud is too loud?" www.windturbinesyndrome.com.

As for the reception I anticipate for this report, I don't flatter myself that it will be greeted with loud hosannas from the wind industry. Keep in mind that wind developers have what is called in science a "conflict of interest." Meaning, their judgment is unduly influenced by money. "It's difficult to get a man to understand something when his salary depends upon his not understanding it," wryly observed Upton Sinclair.[23]

I have no conflict of interest. This research was unfunded, and neither my small village property, my town, nor the Adirondack Park bordering my town is a likely candidate for a wind farm. Is a fondness for bats and other interesting, highly evolved animals a conflict of interest? I wouldn't think so. Admittedly I am distressed to hear about bats dying of internal hemorrhage as they fly near wind turbines,[24] just as I am distressed to hear that people are forced from their homes or endure cognitive impairment of uncertain reversibility in order to remain in the only home they can afford. I have spoken and written earnestly and vigorously about wind developers, because of their stubborn refusal to acknowledge health problems amply documented in this and other studies.[25] Such stonewalling would test the patience of a saint, and I am no saint.

---

[23] Sinclair, Upton. 1935. *I, Candidate for Governor: And How I Got Licked.* Farrar & Rinehart, NY.

[24] Baerwald EF, d'Amours GH, Klug BJ, Barclay RM. 2008. Barotrauma is a significant cause of bat fatalities at wind turbines. Curr Biol 18(16): R695–96. Due to air pressure shifts near moving turbine blades, blood vessels in bats' lungs and abdomen are disrupted, which produces fatal internal hemorrhage.

[25] In anticipation of wind industry blowback, I imagine it may once again publicize that it thinks I think wind turbines cause mad cow disease. I do not and never did. My reply to this canard—now a Pierpont family joke—was published several years ago (www.windturbinesyndrome.com/?p=84). My previous reports and papers on Wind Turbine Syndrome and the wind industry can be found on www.windturbinesyndrome.com.

My hope is that this report will balance the risk-benefit picture of wind turbines more realistically, and help those individuals, such as George Kamperman and Rick James, who are actively promoting noise control criteria that will stem the health and home abandonment problems documented here.

Kamperman and James have convinced me that a single, one-size-fits-all setback distance may not be both protective and fair in all environments with all types of turbines. Even so, it is clear from this study and others that minimum protective distances need to be:

a) greater than 1–1.5 km (3280–4900 ft or 0.62–0.93 mi), at which there were severely affected subjects in this study;

b) greater than 1.6 km (5250 ft or 1 mi), at which there were affected subjects in Dr. Harry's UK study;

c) and, in mountainous terrain, greater than 2–3.5 km (1.24–2.2 mi), at which there were symptomatic subjects in Professor Robyn Phipps's New Zealand study.[26]

Two kilometers, or 1.24 miles, remains the baseline, shortest setback from residences (and hospitals, schools, nursing homes, etc.) that communities should consider. In mountainous terrain, 2 miles (3.2 km) is probably a better guideline. Setbacks may well need to be longer than these minima, as guided by the noise criteria developed by Kamperman and James.

The shorter setbacks currently in use in the USA and elsewhere, 1000–1500 ft (305–457 m), are a convenience and financial advantage for wind developers and leaseholding landowners. They

---

[26] See pp. 31–32 for discussion and references.

have no basis in research on safety and health, and they make no clinical sense.

For those who read this report and recognize their own symptoms, the appropriate medical specialist to consult would be a neurotologist (or otoneurologist), who is an otolaryngologist (ear, nose, and throat doctor) who specializes in balance, the inner ear, and their neurological connections. When I sent this report out for critical review, these were the physicians who recognized a remarkably similar symptom complex from cases familiar to them—such as certain inner-ear pathologies.

To those of you living near turbines and recognizing your own symptoms within these pages: you are not crazy and not fabricating them. Your symptoms are clinically valid—and unnecessary. While wind developers rush headlong into yet more projects, you unfortunates will have to exercise patience as the medical profession catches up with what is ailing you. Meanwhile, my advice is, speak out. In *The Tyranny of Noise*, Robert Alex Baron calls for an end to "our passive acceptance of industry's acoustic waste products."[27]

This will happen only when the suffering refuse to be silenced.

By the time I finished interviewing and moved on to data analysis (February 2008), six of my ten families had moved out of their homes because of turbine-associated symptoms. Three months later (May 2008), when the first draft was complete and I contacted the families for their approval and permission to publish the information on them, two more had moved out because of their turbine-associated symptoms—bringing the total to eight of the ten. The ninth family could not afford to move, but had done extensive renovations in an

---

[27] Baron, Robert Alex. 1970. *The Tyranny of Noise: The World's Most Prevalent Pollution, Who Causes It, How It's Hurting You, and How to Fight It*. St. Martin's Press, New York, p. 12.

effort to keep the noise out. (Renovations, ironically, that made the house worse to live in, since they could no longer heat it properly.) As of this writing, family number ten is struggling to remain in their home.

Behold ten families whose lives have been turned upside down because of the wind industry's acoustic waste products.

Finally, ask yourself why a country doctor practicing in the poorest county in New York State did this study, and not the Centers for Disease Control or some other relevant government agency. It's a fair question and a troubling one. I ask it myself.

It is well known that wind developers target impoverished communities for their wind farms. This explains the "poorest county" part of my question, and likewise why wind turbines quickly became a looming issue in my life four years ago. But it leaves unanswered the part about, "Why did I write this report, and not the government?"

To answer that would of necessity catapult this report (and me) into the treacherous territory of public policy. One would like to think science is not beholden (craven?) to public policy, but that would be naïve, would it not? Moreover, while the scientist in me would like to imagine that I can write this report and remain above the hurly-burly of public policy, I know this, too, is naïve. Wind Turbine Syndrome is an industrial plague. It is man-made and easily fixed. Proper setbacks are the best cure I know of; they do the job just fine. If I could scrawl this on a prescription pad and hand it to my subjects in this report, I would do so. No brilliant scientist needs to discover a new antibiotic or vaccine or sleeping pill to treat it.

Setbacks, however, are not considered matters of public health, but matters of public policy—what is called "politics." And right there is the rub. In the global rush to wind energy there is almost no voice heard for public health repercussions. Where it is heard—at town meetings, on the Internet, in Letters to the Editor, in courtrooms—it is routinely ridiculed. I speak from experience.

Wind energy is being promoted by every state and national government I know of, under intense lobbying by wind development companies generally owned or otherwise capitalized by powerful investment banks which in turn take large tax write-offs and reap large government subsidies for their wind farm projects. These companies turn around and sell carbon credits (green credits). Perhaps this helps explain why no provision is made for clinical caution?

And perhaps this goes some way toward explaining why a pediatrician in rural New York State and a general practitioner in Cornwall, England—along with a handful of rank-and-file, community physicians elsewhere in the UK, USA, Australia, and who knows where else—are the ones funding this research and writing these reports.

Then so be it.

Three poems by Gail Atkinson-Mair, who has lived every page in this book:

> **The Moles**
> You call me to the window, not quite sure,
> "I really get the feeling we've got fewer moles
> —must be the cat." An end to an unending war,
> you grin and raise your glass. You're right. The holes
> that spotty-dicked the grass and made me think

of crazy golf have by some miracle grown rare. I
frown and look away, then crash the dishes in the sink
and fumble, ill at ease. Alarm bells ring—but why?
There's something not quite right today—
a smooth expanse of light rich green and not one
mole hill to be seen; a thousand velvet diggers gone.
We look at one another and although
our mud-filled brains urge us to stay
our guts tell us—it's time to go.

Home
She's like the flies that buzz around inside
the house, alight on window, table, chair
and then take off. She stands, she sits, she looks
around a moment, then she's off. Eyes wide
she searches, checks, then stops. Smoothes hair
from face, swipes dust from books.
She's pulled the plugs and fixtures out,
switched off the mains, "Not there," she said.
She's gone outside and come back in,
It isn't there. You know it's not! I want to shout
and make her stop. The buzzing in her head
will drive her mad. She grabs the radio and plugs it in
then plugs her ears. Her face is grey
"Stop it now," she screams at me, "and make it go away."

My Back Yard
I had to come before I go insane.
The plant you built has side effects: I vomit, weep,
have dizzy spells and I'm depressed. The pain
from pressure in my ears keeps me from sleep—
I wake up drenched, have jitters, palpitations.
Your "silent" noise impairs my concentration—
I think you call that torture.

I no longer have a garden or a view, your
symphony of turbines has drowned the song of nature.
You say you've done what is required by law
but tell me where do people feature?
How old are you, Ms May? Aha, the menopause . . .
We call this problem, "NIMBY," I think you'll find . . .
Damn right, you are. It's not in your back yard—it's mine.

TWO
The REPORT, for clinicians

Abstract

This report documents a consistent and often debilitating complex of symptoms experienced by adults and children while living near large industrial wind turbines (1.5–3 MW). It examines patterns of individual susceptibility and proposes pathophysiologic mechanisms. Symptoms include sleep disturbance, headache, tinnitus, ear pressure, dizziness, vertigo, nausea, visual blurring, tachycardia, irritability, problems with concentration and memory, and panic episodes associated with sensations of internal pulsation or quivering that arise while awake or asleep.

The study is a case series of 10 affected families, with 38 members age <1 to 75, living 305 m to 1.5 km (1000 to 4900 ft) from wind turbines erected since 2004. All competent and available adults and older teens completed a detailed clinical interview about their own and their children's symptoms, sensations, and medical conditions a) before turbines were erected near their homes, b) while living near operating turbines, and c) after leaving their homes or spending a prolonged period away.

Statistically significant risk factors for symptoms during exposure include pre-existing migraine disorder, motion sensitivity, or inner-ear damage (pre-existing tinnitus, hearing loss, or industrial noise exposure). Symptoms are not statistically associated with pre-existing anxiety or other mental health disorders. The symptom complex resembles syndromes caused by vestibular dysfunction. People without known risk factors are also affected.

The proposed pathophysiology posits disturbance to balance and position sense when low frequency noise or vibration stimulates receptors for the balance system (vestibular, somatosensory, or visceral sensory, as well as visual stimulation from moving shadows) in a discordant fashion. Vestibular neural signals are known to affect a variety of brain areas and functions, including spatial awareness, spatial memory, spatial problem-solving, fear, anxiety, autonomic functions, and aversive learning, providing a robust neural framework for the symptom associations in Wind Turbine Syndrome. Further research is needed to prove causes and physiologic mechanisms, establish prevalence, and explore effects in special populations, including children. This and other studies suggest that safe setbacks will be at least 2 km (1.24 mi), and will be longer for larger turbines and in more varied topography.

Introduction and Background

Policy initiatives in the United States and abroad currently encourage the construction of extremely large wind-powered electric generation plants (wind turbines) in rural areas. In its current format, wind electric generation is a variably regulated, multi-billion-dollar-a-year industry. Wind turbines are now commonly placed close to homes. Usual setbacks in New York State, for example, are 305–457 m (1000–1500 ft) from houses.[1] Developer statements and preconstruction modeling lead

---

[1] Town of Ellenburg, NY, wind law: 1000 ft (305 m); Town of Clinton, NY, wind law: 1200 ft (366 m); Town of Martinsburg, NY, wind law: 1500 ft (457 m). For other examples in and outside NY State, see *Wind Energy Development: A Guide for Local Authorities in New York,* New York State Energy Research and Development Authority, October 2002, p. 27. http://text.nyserda.org/programs/pdfs/windguide.pdf.

communities to believe that disturbances from noise and vibration will be negligible or nonexistent.[2–4] Developers assure prospective communities that turbines are no louder than a refrigerator, a library reading room, or the rustling of tree leaves which, they say, easily obscures turbine noise.[5]

Despite these assurances, some people experience significant symptoms after wind turbines are placed in operation near their homes. The purpose of this study is to establish a case definition for the consistent, frequently debilitating, set of symptoms

---

[2] "The GE 1.5 MW wind turbine, which is in use in Fenner, New York, is generally no louder than 50 decibels (dBA) at a distance of 1,000 feet (the closest we would propose siting a turbine to a residence). Governmental and scientific agencies have described 50 dBA as being equivalent to a 'quiet room.' Please keep in mind that these turbines only turn when the wind blows, and the sound of the wind itself is often louder than 50 dBA. Our own experience, and that of many others who live near or have visited the Fenner windfarm, is that the turbines can only be heard when it is otherwise dead quiet, and even then it is very faint, especially at a distance." Letter from Noble Environmental Power, LLC, to residents of Churubusco (Town of Clinton), New York, 7/31/2005.

[3] "Virtually everything with moving parts will make some sound, and wind turbines are no exception. However, well-designed wind turbines are generally quiet in operation, and compared to the noise of road traffic, trains, aircraft, and construction activities, to name but a few, the noise from wind turbines is very low.... Today, an operating wind farm at a distance of 750 to 1,000 feet is no noisier than a kitchen refrigerator or a moderately quiet room." Facts about wind energy and noise. American Wind Energy Association, August 2008, p. 2. www.windturbinesyndrome.com/?p=698.

[4] "In general, wind plants are not noisy, and wind is a good neighbor. Complaints about noise from wind projects are rare, and can usually be satisfactorily resolved." Facts about wind energy and noise. American Wind Energy Association, August 2008, p. 4. www.windturbinesyndrome.com/?p=698.

[5] "Outside the nearest houses, which are at least 300 metres away, and more often further, the sound of a wind turbine generating electricity is likely to be about the same level as noise from a flowing stream about 50–100 metres away or the noise of leaves rustling in a gentle breeze. This is similar to the sound level inside a typical living room with a gas fire switched on, or the reading room of a library or in an unoccupied, quiet, air-conditioned office.... Even when the wind speed increases, it is difficult to detect any increase in turbine sound above the increase in normal background sound, such as the noise the wind itself makes and the rustling of trees." Noise from wind turbines: the facts. British Wind Energy Association, August 2008. www.windturbinesyndrome.com/?p=698.

experienced by people while living near wind turbine installations, and to place this symptom complex within the context of known pathophysiology. A case definition is needed to allow studies of causation, epidemiology, and outcomes to go forward, and to establish adequate community controls.

This set of symptoms stands out in the context of noise control practice. George Kamperman, P.E., INCE Bd. Cert., past member of the acoustics firm Bolt, Beranek and Newman (USA), wrote, "After the first day of digging into the wind turbine noise impact problems in different countries, it became clear that people living within about two miles from 'wind farms' all had similar complaints and health problems. I have never seen this type of phenomenon [in] over fifty plus years of consulting on industrial noise problems. The magnitude of the impact is far above anything I have seen before at such relatively low sound levels. I can see the devastating health impact from wind turbine noise but I can only comment on the physical noise exposure. From my viewpoint we desperately need noise exposure level criteria."[6]

I named this complex of symptoms "Wind Turbine Syndrome" in a preliminary fashion in testimony before the Energy Committee of the New York State Legislature on March 7, 2006. My observation that people can feel vibration or pulsations from wind turbines, and find it disturbing, was quoted in the brief section, "Impacts on Human Health and Well-Being" in the report *Environmental Impacts of Wind-Energy Projects* of the National Academy of Science, published in May 2007. No other medical information was cited in this report. The authors asked for more information to better understand these effects.[7]

---

[6] George Kamperman, personal communication, 2/21/2008. See www.kamperman.com/index.htm.

[7] National Research Council. 2007. *Environmental Impacts of Wind-Energy Projects*. The National Academies Press, Washington, DC. 185 pp, p. 109.

Debates about wind turbine–associated health problems have been dominated to date by noise control engineers, or acousticians, which is problematic in part because the acoustics field at present is dominated by the wind turbine industry,[8] and in part because acousticians are not trained in medicine. A typical approach to wind turbine disturbance complaints, world-wide, is *noise first, symptoms second*: if an acoustician can demonstrate with noise measurements that there is no noise considered significant in a setting, then the symptoms experienced by people in that setting can be, and frequently are, dismissed. This has been the experience of seven of the ten families in this study in the United States, Canada, Ireland, and Italy.[9] At least one developer has put forward the hypothesis that a negative attitude or worry towards turbines is what leads people to be disturbed by turbine noise.[10]

---

[8] George Kamperman, personal communication, 2/23/2008.

[9] A notable exception to this pattern is the physics research and modeling of GP van den Berg, who, as a graduate student and member of the Science Shop for Physics of the University of Groningen in the Netherlands, investigated noise complaints near a windplant and devised new models of atmospheric noise propagation to fit the phenomena he observed. References: 1) van den Berg, GP. 2004. Effects of the wind profile at night on wind turbine sound. J Sound Vib 277: 955–70; 2) van den Berg, GP. 2004. Do wind turbines produce significant low frequency sound levels? 11th International Meeting on Low Frequency Noise and Vibration and Its Control, Maastricht, Netherlands, August 30 to September 1, 8 pp.; 3) van den Berg, GP. 2005. The beat is getting stronger: the effect of atmospheric stability on low frequency modulated sound of wind turbines. J Low Freq Noise Vib Active Contr 24(1): 1–24; 4) van den Berg, GP. 2006. The sound of high winds: the effect of atmospheric stability on wind turbine sound and microphone noise. PhD dissertation, University of Groningen, Netherlands. 177 pp. http://irs.ub.rug.nl/ppn/294294104

[10] "We often use the word 'noise' to refer to 'any unwanted sound.' It's true that wind turbines make sounds … but whether or not those sounds are 'noisy' has a lot to do with who's listening. It's also worth noting that studies have shown [no references provided in source document] that a person's attitude toward a sound—meaning whether it's a 'wanted' or 'unwanted' sound—depends a great deal on what they think and how they feel about the source of the sound. In other words, if someone has a negative attitude to wind turbines, or is worried about them, this will affect how they feel about the sound. However, if someone has a positive attitude toward wind energy, it's very unlikely that the sounds will bother them at all." Wind fact sheet #5: Are modern wind turbines noisy? p. 2. Noble Environmental Power, LLC. www.windturbinesyndrome.com/?p=698.

A reorientation is in order. If people are so disturbed by their headaches, tinnitus, sleeplessness, panic episodes, disrupted children, or memory deficits that they must move or abandon their homes to get away from wind turbine noise and vibration, then that noise and vibration is by definition significant, because the symptoms it causes are significant. The role of an ethical acoustician is to figure out what type and intensity of noise or vibration creates particular symptoms, and to propose effective control measures.

My study subjects make it clear that their problems are caused by noise and vibration. Some symptoms in some subjects are also triggered by moving blade shadows. However, I do not present or analyze noise data in this study, because noise is not my training. (Conversely, symptoms and disease are not the training of acousticians.) I focus on detailed symptomatic descriptions and statistical evaluation of medical susceptibility factors within the study group. Correlating the noise and vibration characteristics of the turbine-exposed homes with the symptoms of the people in the homes is an area ripe for collaboration between medical researchers and independent noise control engineers.

Other than articles on the Internet, there is currently no published research on wind turbine–associated symptoms. A UK physician, Dr. Amanda Harry, whose practice includes patients living near wind turbines, has published online the results of a checklist survey, documenting specific symptoms among 42 adults who identified themselves to her as having problems while living 300 m to 1.6 km (984 ft to 1 mi) from turbines.[11] She found a high prevalence of sleep disturbance, fatigue, headache, migraine, anxiety, depression, tinnitus, hearing loss, and palpitations. Respondents described a similar set of symptoms and many of the same experiences that

---

[11] Harry, Amanda. 2007. Wind turbines, noise, and health. 32 pp. www.windturbine noisehealthhumanrights.com/wtnoise_health_2007_a_barry.pdf

I document in this report, including having to move out of their homes because of symptoms. Respondents were mostly older adults: 42% were age 60 or older, 40% age 45–60, 12% age 30–45, and 5% age 18–30. A biomedical librarian, Barbara Frey, working with this physician and others, has published online a compilation of other personal accounts of symptoms and sensations near wind turbines.[12] These also mirror what I document.

Robyn Phipps, PhD, a New Zealand scientist specializing in health in indoor environments, systematically surveyed residents up to 15 km (9.3 mi) from operating wind turbine installations, asking both positive and negative questions about visual, noise, and vibration experiences.[13] All respondents (614 or 56% of the 1100 households to whom surveys were mailed) lived at least 2 km (1.24 mi) from turbines, with 85% of respondents living 2–3.5 km (1.24–2.2 mi) from turbines and 15% farther away. Among other questions, the survey asked about unpleasant physical sensations from turbine noise, which were experienced by 2.1% of respondents, even at these distances. Forty-one respondents (6.7%) spontaneously telephoned Dr. Phipps to tell her more than was asked on the survey about their distress due to turbine noise and vibration, nearly all (39) with disturbed sleep.[14] Symptoms were not further differentiated in this study, but clearly may occur at distances even greater than 2 km (1.24 mi) from turbines.

Published survey studies have examined residents' reactions to wind turbines relative to modeled noise levels and visibility of

---

[12] Frey, Barbara J, and Hadden, Peter J. 2007. Noise radiation from wind turbines installed near homes: effects on health. 137 pp. www.windturbinenoisehealthhumanrights.com/wtnhhr_june2007.pdf.

[13] Phipps, Robyn. 2007. Evidence of Dr. Robyn Phipps, in the matter of Moturimu wind farm application heard before the Joint Commissioners, March 8–26. Palmerston North, New Zealand. 43 pp. www.wind-watch.org/documents/wp-content/uploads/phipps-moturimutestimony.pdf.

[14] Phipps 2007.

turbines in Sweden[15-17] and the Netherlands.[18-20] The study in the Netherlands included questions on health, though not of sufficient power to make any statements on health other than the correspondence between sleep disturbance and modeled noise (see below, Discussion). Both sets of studies, the Swedish and Dutch, have findings that could contribute to the rational setting of noise limits near wind turbines (see Discussion).

With regard to official opinion, the National Academy of Medicine in France recommended in 2005 that industrial wind turbines be sited at least 1.5 km (0.93 mi) from human habitation due to health effects of low frequency noise produced by the turbines.[21]

Current wind turbines have three airfoil-shaped rotor blades attached by a hub to gears and a generator, which are housed in a bus-sized box (nacelle) at the top of a nearly cylindrical, hollow

---

[15] Pedersen E, Persson Waye K. 2004. Perceptions and annoyance due to wind turbine noise: a dose-response relationship. J Acoust Soc Am 116(6): 3460–70.

[16] Pedersen E. 2007. Human response to wind turbine noise: perception, annoyance and moderating factors. PhD dissertation, Occupational and Environmental Medicine, Department of Public Health and Community Medicine, Göteborg University, Göteborg, Sweden. 86 pp.

[17] Pedersen E, Persson Waye K. 2007. Wind turbine noise, annoyance and self-reported health and wellbeing in different living environments. Occup Environ Med 64(7): 480–86.

[18] Pedersen E, Bouma J, Bakker R, van den Berg GP. 2008. Response to wind turbine noise in the Netherlands. J Acoust Soc Am 123(5): 3536 (abstract).

[19] van den Berg GP, Pedersen E, Bakker R, Bouma J. 2008. Wind farm aural and visual impact in the Netherlands. J Acoust Soc Am 123(5): 3682 (abstract).

[20] van den Berg GP, Pedersen E, Bouma J, Bakker R. 2008. Project WINDFARMperception: visual and acoustic impact of wind turbine farms on residents. Final report, June 3. 63 pp. Summary: http://umcg.wewi.eldoc.ub.rug.nl/FILES/root/Rapporten/2008/WINDFARMperception/WFp-final-summary.pdf. Entire report: https://dspace.hh.se/dspace/bitstream/2082/2176/1/WFp-final.pdf.

[21] Académie nationale de médecine de France. 2006. "Le retentissement du fonctionnement des éoliennes sur la santé de l'homme, le Rapport, ses Annexes et les Recommandations de l'Académie nationale de médecine, 3/14/2006." 17 pp. www.academie-medecine.fr/sites_thematiques/EOLIENNES/chouard_rapp_14mars_2006.htm.

steel tower. The nacelle is rotated mechanically to face the blades into the wind. The blades spin upwind of the tower. The tower is anchored in a steel-reinforced concrete foundation. Turbine heights in this study were 100 to 135 m (328 to 443 ft) with hub heights 59 to 90 m (194 to 295 ft) and blade lengths 33 to 45 m (108 to 148 ft). Individual turbine powers were 1.5 to 3 MW. Clusters contained from 8 to 45 individual turbines (see Table 1B).

In this study, participants from all families described good and bad symptomatic periods correlated with particular sounds from the turbine installations, rate of turbine spin, or whether the turbines were turned towards, away from, or sideways relative to their homes. All participants identified wind directions and intensities that exacerbated their problems and others that brought relief. Many subjects described a quality of invasiveness in wind turbine noise, more disturbing than other noises like trains. Some stated that the noise wouldn't sound loud to people who did not live with it, or that noises described with benign-sounding terms like "swish" or "hum" were in reality very disturbing. Several were disturbed specifically by shadow flicker, which is the flashing of light in a room as the slanting sun shines through moving turbine blades, or the repetitive movement of the shadows across yards and walls. (These observations are documented in the narrative data of the CASE HISTORIES.)

Wind turbines generate sound across the spectrum from the infrasonic to the ultrasonic,[22] and also produce ground-borne or seismic vibration.[23] "In the broadest sense, a sound wave is any disturbance that is propagated in an elastic medium, which may be

---

[22] van den Berg 2004a.

[23] Styles P, Stimpson I, Toon S, England R, and Wright M. 2005. Microseismic and infrasound monitoring of low frequency noise and vibrations from wind farms: recommendations on the siting of wind farms in the vicinity of Eskdalemuir, Scotland. 125 pp. www.esci.keele.ac.uk/geophysics/News/windfarm_monitoring.html

a gas, a liquid, or a solid. Ultrasonic, sonic, and infrasonic waves are included in this definition.... Sonic waves [are] those waves that can be perceived by the hearing sense of the human being. Noise is defined as any perceived sound that is objectionable to a human being."[24]

Following standard usage in noise literature, I use the word *vibration* to refer to disturbances in solid media, such as the ground, house structures, or the human body. When air-borne sound waves of particular energy (power) and frequency meet a solid object, they may set the object vibrating. Conversely, a vibrating solid object, such as the strings on a violin, can create sound waves in air. There is energy transfer in both directions between air-borne or fluid-borne sound waves and the vibration of solids. When I talk about noise and vibration together, I am referring to this continuum of mechanical energy in the air and solids.

Energy in either form (sound or vibration) can impinge on the human body, and there may be multiple exchanges between air and solids in the path between a source and a human. The tissues of humans and other animals are semi-liquid to varying degrees, and have fluid-filled and air-filled spaces within them, as well as solid structures like bones. As an example of such energy transfer, a sound wave in the air, encountering a house, may set up vibrations in the structure of the house. These vibrations, in walls or windows, may set up air pressure (sound) waves in rooms, which can in turn transmit mechanical energy to the tympanic membrane and middle ear, to the airways and lungs, and to body surfaces. Alternatively, vibrations in house structures or the ground may transmit energy directly to the body by solid-to-solid contact and be conducted through the body by bone conduction.

---

[24] Beranek LL. 2006. Basic acoustical quantities: levels and decibels. Chapter 1 in *Noise and Vibration Control and Engineering: Principles and Applications*, ed. Ver IL, Beranek LL, pp. 1–24. John Wiley & Sons, Hoboken, NJ. p. 1.

All parts of the body (and indeed all objects) have specific resonance frequencies, meaning that *particular frequencies or wavelengths of sound will be amplified in that body part.*[25] If the wavelength of a sound or its harmonic matches the dimensions of a room, it may set up standing waves in the room with places where the intersecting, reverberating sound waves reinforce each other. Resonance also occurs inside air-filled body cavities such as the lungs, trachea, pharynx, middle ear, mastoid, and gastrointestinal tract. The elasticity of the walls and density of the contents of these spaces affect the dynamics of sound waves inside them. The orbits (bones surrounding the eyes) and cranial vault (braincase) are also resonance chambers, because of the lower density of their contents compared to the bones that surround them. There are also vibratory resonance patterns along the spine (which is elastic), including a resonance involving the movement of the head relative to the shoulders. Von Gierke[26,27] and Rasmussen[28] have described the resonant frequencies of different parts of the human body.

Noise intensity is measured in decibels (dB), a logarithmic scale of sound pressure amplitude. Single noise measurements or integrated measurements over time combine the energies of a range of frequencies into a single number, as defined by the filter or weighting network used during the measurement. The A-weighting

---

[25] Hedge, Alan. 2007. Department of Design and Environmental Analysis, Cornell University. Syllabus/lecture notes for DEA 350: Whole-body vibration (January), found at http://ergo.human.cornell.edu/studentdownloads/DEA325pdfs/Human%20Vibration.pdf

[26] von Gierke HE, Parker DE. 1994. Differences in otolith and abdominal viscera graviceptor dynamics: implications for motion sickness and perceived body position. Aviat Space Environ Med 65(8): 747–51.

[27] von Gierke HE. 1971. Biodynamic models and their applications. J Acoust Soc Am 50(6): 1397–413.

[28] Rasmussen G. 1982. Human body vibration exposure and its measurement. Bruel and Kjaer Technical Paper No. 1, Naerum, Denmark. Abstract: Rasmussen G. 1983. Human body vibration exposure and its measurement. J Acoust Soc Am 73(6): 2229.

network is the most common in studies of community noise. It is designed to duplicate the frequency response of human hearing for air-borne sounds entering through the outer and middle ear. A-weighting slightly augments the contributions of sounds in the 1000 to 6000 Hz range (from C two octaves above middle C, key 64 on the piano, to F# above the highest note on the piano), and progressively reduces the contributions of lower frequencies below about 800 Hz (G-G# 1½ octaves above middle C, keys 59–60). At 100 Hz, where the human inner-ear vestibular organ has a peak response to vibration[29] (G-G# 1½ octaves below middle C, keys 23–24), A-weighting reduces sound measurement by a factor of 1000 (30 dB). At 31 Hz (B, the second-to-bottom white key, key 3), A-weighting reduces sound measurement by a factor of 10,000 (40 dB). Thus A-weighting preferentially captures the high sounds used in language recognition, to which the human cochlea and outer and middle ear are indeed very sensitive, but reduces the contribution of mid- and lower-range audible sounds, as well as infrasound (defined as 20 Hz and below).

Linear (lin) measurements use no weighting network, so the frequency responses are limited by other aspects of the system, such as microphone sensitivity. Linear measurements may capture low frequency sounds but are not standardized—different sound level meters yield different results. As a result, the standardized and commonly available C-weighting network is preferred for measuring environmental noise with low frequency components, such as noise from wind turbines. The C-weighting network has a flat response (meaning that it does not reduce or enhance the contributions of different frequencies) over the audible frequency range and a well-defined decreasing response below 31 Hz.

---

[29] Todd NPMc, Rosengren SM, Colebatch JG. 2008. Tuning and sensitivity of the human vestibular system to low-frequency vibration. Neurosci Lett 444: 36–41.

One third (1/3) octave band studies are used to describe sound pressure levels by frequency, and are presented as a graph rather than a single number. One third (1/3) octave bands can also be measured linearly or with weighting networks.

Methods

The study design is a case series of affected families, interviewed by telephone. I used a broad-based, structured interview including a narrative account, symptom checklist, past medical and psychiatric history, personal and social history, selected elements of family history, and review of systems. This is the "history" in the standard physician's "history and physical," with specific questions oriented towards the problems in question. The core of the syndrome consists of symptoms such as sleep disturbance, headache, tinnitus, dizziness, nausea, anxiety, concentration problems, and others which are typically diagnosed by medical history more than physical exam.

Limited medical records were provided by the adults of families A and B (A1, A2, B1, B2) and by a young man in family C (C4). I requested records for all families through F, but since no more were forthcoming, I stopped asking, and pursued those parts of the study not dependent on physical examination or test results, and for which I had a uniform study tool, the interview.

The study design includes comparison groups in two ways: 1) I obtained information for each symptom before exposure, during exposure, and away from or after the end of exposure, so that each subject acted as his or her own control in the "natural experiment" of living in a home under a certain set of conditions, having wind turbines added to those conditions, and then moving or going away and again experiencing an environment without turbines. Subjects also noted how their symptom intensity varied in concert with the type and loudness of noise, the direction turbine blades were turned, the rate of spin, or the presence or absence of shadow flicker. A positive symptom is one that emerged from the within-subject comparison as distinctly worse during exposure than before or after (generally both). For example, a subject was considered to have headaches due to turbine exposure only if his (her) headaches were more frequent, severe, or longer-lasting during turbine exposure than his own headaches before being exposed to turbines and after ending the exposure. 2) I obtained information on all household members, not only the most affected, so that I could compare more affected to less affected subjects, all of whom were exposed, to evaluate individual risk factors with regard to age, sex, and underlying health conditions.

Families were selected to conform to all of the following: 1) severity of symptoms of at least one family member; 2) presence of a "post-exposure" condition, in which the family had either left the affected home or spent periods of time away; 3) quality of observation, memory, and expression, so that interviewed people were able to state clearly, consistently, and in detail what had happened to them under what conditions and at what time (all but one individual were native English speakers); 4) residence near recently erected turbines (placed in operation 2004–2007); 5) short time span between moving out and the interview, if exposure had already ended (six weeks was the maximum); and 6) family actions in response to turbine noise showing how serious and debilitating the symptoms were (moving out, purchasing a second home, leaving home for months, renovating house, sleeping in root cellar).

Most families who met these criteria and were willing to be interviewed lived outside the United States. In the course of the study, I received direct evidence that participation by Americans was limited by non-medical factors such as turbine leases or neighbor contracts prohibiting criticism, court decisions restricting criticism of turbine projects, and community relationships. The same factors are likely, in future, to affect other studies of wind turbine noise effects in the United States, with the potential to introduce significant bias into any population-based study.

Moving is an economic hardship for all the families in the study. All own (or owned) their homes, but only three of the eight families who have left their homes have sold them: one to the utility operating the turbines, one to a buyer introduced to the family by the turbine owner, and one to an independent buyer. Three families do not have their homes for sale because the properties include farmland which they farm or lease out. These families have rented additional houses in nearby villages for living and sleeping, though they can ill afford it. The remaining two families who have left their homes are trying to sell the homes, but have not been successful. One of the two families that have not moved is trying to sell their home so they can move. The tenth family has not moved and is not at this point trying to sell the home.

Though not by design, each case household consisted of a married couple or a married couple with children. One family included an older parent. I interviewed both members of each couple except for one man with dementia, and I interviewed the older parent together with her daughter-in-law. I directly interviewed three out of the four subjects in the 16- to 21-year-old age group; the fourth did not make himself available. Child data are otherwise derived from the parent interviews.

I audio-recorded the interviews for the first two families (C and D, in 2006) as I was developing the interview protocol, but after that noted answers directly on an interview form, writing down distinctive or critical observations and symptom descriptions verbatim. Because of subject time constraints, I also audio-recorded the final family (J, in 2008). Subjects who were recorded gave their permission verbally at the beginning of the interview. I made a confidentiality statement and informed subjects that they would have the opportunity to review the data presented about them prior to publication. Follow-up interviews were done with families C, D, and G. Other families have kept in touch by email and telephone about further developments. All ten families have reviewed the information presented about them and signed permission for anonymous publication.

I use simple statistical tests (2x2 χ^2) to examine associations among symptoms and between pre-existing conditions and symptoms during exposure.[30] Degrees of freedom (df) are 2 for all the χ^2 results in this report. Children were excluded from the analysis of adult symptoms if no child younger than a certain age had the symptom in question. Study children were categorized into developmental-age blocks (see Table 1C). When I excluded children from an analysis, I excluded all the children in that age block and below. Excluding children from adult symptom analyses avoided inflating the no symptom/absent pre-existing condition box of the 2x2 χ^2 contingency tables, which could artificially increase the χ^2 value.

Results

I interviewed 23 adult and teenage members of 10 families, collecting information on all 38 adult, teen, and child family members. One family member was a baby born a few days before the family (A) moved out, so there are no data for this child on sleep or behavior during exposure (which was in utero). Thus the sample size of subjects for whom we have information about experiences or behavior during exposure is 37.

---

[30] Sokal RR, Rohlf FJ. 1969. *Biometry.* W. H. Freeman, San Francisco.

Residence status and family composition are detailed in Table 1A; turbine, terrain, and house characteristics in Table 1B; and the age and sex distribution of subjects in Table 1C. Twenty subjects were male and 18 female, ranging in age from <1 to 75. Seventeen subjects were age 21 and below, and 21 subjects were age 32 and above. There is a gap in the 20's and a preponderance of subjects in their 50's. Wind turbine brands to which study subjects were exposed included Gamesa, General Electric, Repower, Bonus (Siemens), and Vestas.

Individual accounts of baseline health status and pre-exposure, during exposure, and post-exposure symptoms or absence of symptoms are presented in the CASE HISTORIES for families A through J, with a separate sub-table (A1, A2, A3, etc.) for each individual. I encourage the reader to read these, because they highlight the before-during-after comparisons for each person, show how the symptoms fit together for individuals, reveal family patterns, and provide subjects' own words for what they feel and detect. When individuals are referred to in the text, the letter and number in parentheses (e.g., A1, C2) refers to the CASE HISTORY table in which that subject's information is found.

Baseline conditions
Eight adult subjects had current or history of serious medical illness, including lupus (1), breast cancer (2), diabetes (1), coronary artery disease (2), hypertension (1), atrial fibrillation with anticoagulation (1), Parkinson's disease (1), ulcer (1), and fibromyalgia (2). Two were male (age 56–64) and six female (age 51–75). Other past and current medical illnesses are listed in Table 2. Four subjects smoked at the beginning of exposure, and five others had smoked in the past (Table 2). There were no seriously ill children in the sample.

Seven subjects had histories of mental health disorders including depression, anxiety, post-traumatic stress disorder (PTSD), and bipolar disorder. Three were male (age 42–56) and four female (age 32–64). One of these men (age 56) also had Alzheimer's disease. There were no children with mental health disorders or developmental disabilities in this sample.

Eight subjects had pre-existing migraine disorder (including two with previous severe sporadic headaches that I interpreted as migraine). Four were male (age 19–42) and four female (age 12–42). An additional seven subjects, age <1 to 17, were children of migraineurs who had not experienced migraines themselves at baseline.

Eight subjects had permanent hearing impairments, defined subjectively or objectively, including mild losses, losses limited to one ear, or impairments of binaural processing. Six were male (age 32–64) and two female (age 51–57).

Six subjects had continuous tinnitus or a history of multiple, discrete episodes of tinnitus prior to exposure. Four were male (age 19–64) and two female (age 33–57).

Twelve subjects had significant previous noise exposure, defined as working in noisy industrial or construction settings; working on or in a diesel boat, truck, bus, farm equipment, or aircraft; a military tour of duty; or operating lawn mowers and chain saws for work. Not included were home or sporadic use of lawn mowers and chain saws, commuting by train or airplane, urban living in general, or playing or listening to music. Nine of the noise-exposed subjects were male (age 19–64) and three female (age 33–53).

Eighteen subjects were known to be motion sensitive prior to exposure, as defined by carsickness as a child or adult, any episode of seasickness, or a history of two or more episodes of vertigo. Ten were male (age 6–64) and eight female (age 12–57).

Table 1A: Cases: personal attributes

Case	Country	# in household	# interviewed	Ages†	Head of household occupations	Residence status
A	Canada	4	2	33, 32, 2½, 2 months	Fisherman, accountant	Moved to a rented house in nearby village 6 months after renovating their own home, which is vacant. Land they own continues to be leased to a farmer.
B*	Canada	3	3	55, 53, 19	Fisherman, homemaker	Moved to a rented house in nearby village. Home is vacant. Land they own, which has been in the family for over a century, continues to be leased to a farmer.
C	Canada	8	3	45, 42, 21, 19, 15, 12, 9, 5	Fisherman, homemaker	Family divided and moved in with extended family members. Home, built 24 years before by husband on land in family for over a century, is vacant and for sale.
D	Canada	2	2	64, 64	Retired/disabled, home health aide	Occupied home, purchased second house in village 25 miles away during study. Sold home and moved after study completed.
E	Canada	2	1	56, 56	Retired/disabled, teacher	Moved to a newly purchased house in a nearby village after turbine utility bought their home and property.

Report for Clinicians 45

Case	Country	# in household	# interviewed	Ages†	Head of household occupations	Residence status
F	UK	4	4	51, 42, 17, 75**	Farmer, nurse midwife	Rented house in nearby village and continue to use farm and home office during day.
G	Ireland	6	2	35, 32, 6, 5, 2, 8 months	Computer programmer, homemaker	Under pressure from family, turbine owner arranged purchase at 30% below pre-turbine value.
H	Ireland	3	2	57, 52, 8	Milk truck driver, homemaker	Family occupies home. Significant renovations made in attempt to exclude noise.
I	Italy	2	2	59, 52	Professional gardener, teacher	Occupied newly built home during study but wife spent months away due to symptoms. Moved out after study completed, leaving home vacant and for sale.
J	USA	4	2	49, 47, 13, 8	Physician, nurse	Family occupies home.

*Families A and B are related and own separate homes on the same property.
**Grandmother living in different house on same property did not move away.
†Underlined ages indicate interviewees.

Table 1B: Cases: physical attributes

Case	Distance to closest turbine	# turbines	MW per turbine	Year placed in operation	Hub height	Total height	Terrain	Configuration of turbines	House construction
A	1000 m (3281 ft)	10	3	2007	90 m	135 m	Hilly with rocky ridges	10 in line point at house at hub level	Wood frame
B*	1000 m (3281 ft)	10	3	2007	90 m	135 m	Hilly with rocky ridges	10 in line point at house at hub level	Wood frame
C	305 m (1000 ft)	17	1.8	2004–05	80 m	125 m	Rocky peninsula	On three sides	Wood frame
D	548 m (1798 ft)	22	1.8	2006	78 m	117 m	Flat farmland	Group on one side	Wood frame
E	423 m (1388 ft)	45	1.5	2006	87 m	120 m	Flat farmland, swamp	On three sides	Brick with stone front
F	930 m (3051 ft)	8	2	2006	59 m	100 m	Flat farmland	5 in line point at house	Brick on cement slab
G	596 m (1955 ft)	32	3	2006	80 m	125 m	Rocky hills	Above house on three sides	Stone cottage, walls 60 cm thick
H	1500 m (4921 ft)	11	2.3	2005	80 m	121 m	Rocky hills	Above house on three sides	Stone cottage, cement slab
I	875 m (2871 ft)	10	2	2006	78 m	121 m	Rocky hills	Across valley at higher elevation	Stone and brick, walls 50 cm thick
J	732 m (2400 ft)	40	2	2007	80 m	123 m	Ridges and valleys	6 in L-shape above house on two sides	Wood frame

*Families A and B are related and own separate homes on the same property.

Table 1C: Cases: demographics

Age	Male	Female	Total
<1	1	1	2
1–3	1	1	2
4–6	2	1	3
7–11	3	0	3
12–15	1	2	3
16–21	2	2	4
22–29	0	0	0
30–39	2	2	4
40–49	3	2	5
50–59	4	5	9
60–69	1	1	2
70–79	0	1	1
Totals	**20**	**18**	**38**

The subjects' baseline conditions are summarized in Table 3.

Seven subjects had a remembered history of a single concussion, and none had a history of a more severe head injury. Six were male (age 19–59) and one female (age 12). I did not collect information on whiplash injury.

Core symptoms
Core symptoms are defined as 1) common and widely described by study participants, 2) closely linked in time and space to turbine exposure, and 3) amenable to diagnosis by medical history. Core symptoms include sleep disturbance, headache, tinnitus, other ear and hearing sensations, disturbances to balance and equilibrium, nausea, anxiety, irritability, energy loss, motivation loss, and disturbances to memory and concentration.

An additional core symptom is a new type of internal or visceral sensation which has no name in the medical lexicon. Subjects struggled to explain these sensations, often apologizing for how strange their words sounded. A physician subject called it "feeling jittery inside" or "internal quivering." Other subjects chose similar words, while others talked about feeling pulsation or beating inside. The physical sensations of quivering, jitteriness, or pulsation are accompanied by acute anxiety, fearfulness, or agitation, irritability, sleep disturbance (since the symptom arises during sleep or wakefulness), and episodes of tachycardia. I call this sensation and accompanying symptoms *Visceral Vibratory Vestibular Disturbance* (VVVD). It is described further below.

Core symptoms are closely correlated with exposure, including being at home, the direction and strength of the wind, whether turbines are facing the home, and the presence of moving blade shadows. Core symptoms all resolve immediately or within hours away from the turbines, with the exception of disturbances of concentration and memory, which resolved immediately in some cases or improved over weeks to months in others.

Core symptoms are summarized in Table 3.

Sleep disturbance. Thirty-two subjects (17 males age 2–64 and 15 females age 2–75) had disturbed sleep. Types of sleep disturbance included: difficulty getting to sleep, frequent or prolonged awakening by turbine noise, frequent or prolonged awakening by awakened children, night terrors (both 2½-year-olds, B3 and G5), nocturnal enuresis (one 5-year-old girl, G4), nocturia (six women age 42–75 and one man age 64; B2, C2, E2, F2, F4, H2, D1), excessive movement during sleep (one 8-year-old boy, H3), excessive nighttime fears (two 5-year-olds, a girl and a boy, C8 and G4), and abrupt arousals from sleep in states of fear and alarm (four women age 42–57; C2, F2, H2, I2). Other adults, though not fearful when they woke up, awoke with physical symptoms similar to their daytime symptoms of anxiety/agitation/internal quivering (three men age 42–64 and two women age 32–53; D1, F1, J1, B2, G2). Four people slept well, including the one infant (G6), a 19-year-old woman (B3), a 47-year-old woman (J2) and her 8-year-old son (J4). It was unclear whether a 56-year-old man with dementia, bipolar disorder, Parkinson's disease, and disturbed sleep at baseline (E1) slept worse than usual or not.

With three exceptions, all types of sleep disturbance resolved immediately whenever subjects slept away from their turbine-exposed homes, including the adult nocturia and the 5-year-old's nocturnal enuresis. A 49-year-old man with a pre-existing sleep disturbance (J1) took two nights to get back to his baseline, and a 45-year-old man (C1) and a 42-year-old man (F1) did not improve all the way to baseline; this was thought to be due to coexisting depression after abandoning their homes.

Table 2: Past and current serious medical illness

	Adult (>22 yo) (n=21)		Child/youth (0–21 yo) (n=17)	
	Male	Female	Male	Female
Breast cancer		2		
Skin cancer	1			
Lupus		1		
Diabetes	1			
Polycystic ovarian syndrome		1		
Coronary artery disease	1	1		
Atrial fibrillation with anticoagulation		1		
Other arrhythmias	1	1		
Hypertension—present		1		
Hypertension—past or pregnancy		2		
Parkinson's disease	1			
Diplopia		1		
Renal function impairment	1			
Ulcer—past	1			
Gastroesophageal reflux	2	3		
Irritable bowel syndrome	1	1		
Fibromyalgia		2		
Osteoarthritis	1	1		
Back pain	2	1	1	
Other joint pain	1			
Asthma	2	2		1
Eczema		1	1	
Frequent/chronic otitis media—present			1	1
Frequent/chronic otitis media—past		1	2	1
Smoking—present	3	1		
Smoking—past	3	1	1	

Table 3: Baseline conditions and core symptom occurrence*

	Total	Male	Ages	Female	Ages	N**	% of sample
Baseline Conditions							
Serious medical illness†	8	2	56–64	6	51–75	38	21
Mental health disorders‡	7	3	42–56	4	32–64	34	21
Migraine disorder	8	4	19–42	4	12–42	34	24
Hearing impairments	8	6	32–64	2	51–57	34	24
Pre-existing tinnitus	6	4	19–64	2	33–57	24	25
Previous noise exposure	12	9	19–64	3	33–53	24	38
Motion sensitivity	18	10	6–64	8	12–57	34	53
Core Symptoms							
Sleep disturbance	32	17	2–64	15	2–75	36	89
Headache	19	8	6–55	11	12–57	34	56
VVVD◊	14	6	32–64	8	32–75	21	67
Dizziness, vertigo, unsteadiness	16	7	19–64	9	12–64	27	59
Tinnitus	14	9	19–64	5	33–57	24	58
Ear pressure or pain	11	6	2–25	5	19–57	36	30
External auditory canal sensation	5	2	42–55	3	52–75	34	15
Memory and concentration deficits (salient+mild/vague)	28	15	6–64	13	5–57	30	93
Irritability, anger	28	15	2–64	13	2–64	37	76
Fatigue, loss of motivation	27	14	2–64	13	2–75	36	75

*A symptom during exposure is defined as distinctly worse for that individual during exposure compared to before and/or after exposure.
**N=number of subjects in which it was possible to know about the condition or symptom, given age and other specific limitations (see p. 41 and subsequent text).
†See p. 42 and Table 2.
‡See p. 42 and subsequent text for definitions of this and other conditions and symptoms.
◊Visceral Vibratory Vestibular Disturbance: See pp. 48 and 55ff.

Headache. Nineteen subjects experienced headaches that were increased in frequency, intensity, and/or duration compared to baseline for that person. Eight were male (age 6–55) and eleven female (age 12–57). Eight had pre-existing migraine (C2, C3, C4, C5, C6, F1, G1, G2). Two women (one a migraineur, one not; C2, E2) had severe headaches provoked by shadow flicker. All other exposure-related headaches were triggered by noise alone. Recovery from headaches generally took several hours after the exposure ended.

Headache risk factors were examined in a subset of the study group that included all subjects age 5 and older (N=34), since the younger children in the study (age <1 to 2) were not reliable sources of information on headache. The occurrence of unusually severe or frequent headaches during exposure was significantly associated with pre-existing migraine disorder ($\chi^2 = 8.26$, $p = 0.004$). All 8 subjects with pre-existing migraine experienced headaches that were unusually intense, frequent, or prolonged compared to their baseline headaches. Of the 26 subjects without pre-existing migraine, 11 also experienced unusual or severe headaches during exposure. Two of these were children of migraineurs not known to have migraine themselves (a girl age 17 and a boy age 6; F3, G3). All children or teens (through age 21) who had headaches during exposure were migraineurs or children of migraineurs.

Once migraine was factored out as a risk factor, 9 of 17 subjects over age 22 without a history of migraine still had headaches of increased intensity, duration, or frequency during exposure to turbines. I found no significant correlation within this group between headache and the presence of serious underlying medical illness ($\chi^2 = 0.486$, $p = 0.486$), present or past mental health disorder ($\chi^2 = 0.476$, $p = 0.490$), tinnitus or hearing loss at baseline, motion sensitivity at baseline, or tinnitus, disequilibrium, or VVVD during exposure.

In summary, a little more than half (19) of the 34 study participants age 5 and older experienced unusually severe headaches during exposure. Migraine was a statistically significant risk factor but was present in fewer than half (8) of the 19 subjects with worsened headache. Children and teens up to age 21 with headaches either had known migraine or were the children of migraineurs. Nine of the 19 headache subjects were adults without clear risk factors, showing that while people with migraine are more likely to have headaches of unusual intensity, duration, or frequency around turbines, so can other adults without identified risk factors.

Ears, hearing, and tinnitus. Fourteen subjects (nine males age 19–64 and five females age 33–57) experienced tinnitus that was new or worse in severity or duration than at baseline. For two men (age 55 and 64; B1, D1), the tinnitus at times interfered with their ability to understand conversation. Four of the 14 subjects experienced particularly disturbing kinds of tinnitus or noise which was perceived to be inside the head (two men age 42, 55, and two women age 52, 57; B1, F1, H2, I2). This sensation was painful for two subjects. Tinnitus tended to resolve over several hours after exposure ended.

Tinnitus risk factors were examined in subjects age 16 and older, since the youngest person with tinnitus was in this age group. The subject with dementia (E1) was excluded, since there was no information on his hearing status or tinnitus. Sample size was 24 subjects. The occurrence of new or worsened tinnitus in the presence of turbines was significantly correlated with previous noise exposure ($\chi^2 = 6.17$, $p = 0.013$), tinnitus prior to exposure ($\chi^2 = 5.71$, $p = 0.017$), and baseline hearing loss ($\chi^2 = 4.20$, $p = 0.040$). New or worsened tinnitus during exposure was strongly correlated with ear popping, ear pressure, or ear pain during exposure ($\chi^2 = 7.11$, $p = 0.008$), and weakly correlated with dizziness/disequilibrium during exposure ($\chi^2 = 3.70$, $p = 0.054$). Tinnitus during exposure did not show a significant relationship with pre-existing migraine or motion sensitivity, or with headache or VVVD during exposure.

Eleven subjects during exposure experienced ear popping, ear or mastoid area pressure, ear pain without infection, or a sensation that the eardrum was moving but not producing a sensation of sound (six males age 2–55 and five females age 19–57). The 2½-year-old (A3) pulled on his ears and got cranky repeatedly at the same time as his grandmother's (B2) exacerbations of headache, tinnitus, and ear pain. Correlations with tinnitus during exposure are described above. Five subjects experienced tickling, blowing, or undefined sensations in the external auditory canal, or increased wax production (two men age 42, 55, and three women age 52–75).

Individual subjects noticed changes in their hearing or auditory processing. A 33-year-old woman (A2) had progressively worsening tinnitus during her five months of exposure. After she moved away, the tinnitus resolved and she noticed she had a new difficulty understanding conversation in a noisy room, now needing to watch the speaker's face carefully. Her son (A3, the 2½-year-old who pulled on his ears and got cranky, above) did not confuse sounds before exposure, but began to do so during exposure, and continued to do so at the time I interviewed his mother six weeks after the exposure ended. The child's language development was otherwise good. A 42-year-old woman (C2) had tinnitus throughout her 21-month exposure period without subjective hearing changes. After she moved and the tinnitus resolved, she noted hyperacusis. A 32-year-old woman (G2) experienced hyperacusis during exposure, but no tinnitus. The hyperacusis resolved after the family moved.

Balance and equilibrium. Sixteen subjects (seven males age 19–64 and nine females age 12–64) experienced disturbance to their balance or sense of equilibrium during exposure, describing dizziness, light-headedness, unsteadiness, or spinning sensations. One of them, a 42-year-old woman (C2), described how a friend, sitting next to her in her turbine-exposed home, remarked how her (C2's) eyes appeared to be bouncing back and forth (nystagmus). Ten of these 16 subjects also experienced nausea during exposure to turbines, during or separate from dizziness. No children under the age of 12 had symptoms of dizziness, disequilibrium, or nausea during exposure, except for the usual nausea of acute gastrointestinal and other infections.

Risk factors for dizziness/disequilibrium in the presence of turbines were analyzed using subjects age 12 and up, since this was the youngest age child with this type of symptom. The subject with Parkinson's disease and dementia (E1) was excluded because his baseline balance problems and inability to express himself made it hard for his wife (the informant) to tell if he had worsened symptoms during exposure or not. The remaining sample was 27 subjects. Disequilibrium during exposure was significantly correlated with headaches during exposure ($\chi^2 = 5.08$, $p = 0.024$) and baseline motion sensitivity ($\chi^2 = 4.20$, $p = 0.040$). Disequilibrium during exposure is weakly correlated with tinnitus during exposure ($\chi^2 = 3.70$, $p = 0.054$). (Inspection of the data shows that these are primarily ataxic (unsteady) subjects.) Dizziness/disequilibrium during exposure was not correlated with VVVD or ear popping/pressure/pain during exposure, pre-existing migraine disorder, previous noise exposure, or prior tinnitus or hearing loss.

Internal quivering, vibration, or pulsation. Eleven adult subjects described these uncomfortable, unfamiliar, and hard-to-explain sensations:

- Dr. J (J1, age 49) described "internal quivering" as part of the "jittery feeling" he has when the turbines are turning fast.

- Mrs. I (I2, age 52) said the noise inside her house is "low, pulsating, almost a vibration," not shut out by earplugs. She gets a sensation inside her chest like "pins and needles" and chest tightness on awakening at night to noise. "It affects my body—this is the feeling I get when I say I'm agitated or jittery. It's this that gives me pressure or ringing in my ears." "A feeling someone has invaded not only my health and my territory, but my body."

- Mrs. H (H2, age 57) described a pulsation that prevented sleep from the "unnatural" noise from the turbines.

- Mr. G (G1, age 35) described feeling disoriented and "very strange" in certain parts of the house where he could "feel rumbling." If he did not move quickly away from these locations, the feeling would progress to nausea. He described the noise as "at times very invasive. Train noise has a different quality, and is not invasive."

- Mrs. G (G2, age 32) felt disoriented, "light-headed," dizzy, and nauseated in her garden and in specific parts of the house where she detected vibration. She felt her body vibrating "inside," but when she put her hand on walls, windows, or objects, they did not seem to be vibrating.

- Mrs. F (F2, age 51) described a physical sensation of noise "like a heavy rock concert," saying the "hum makes you feel sick."

- Mrs. E (E2, age 56), when supine, felt a "ticking" or "pulsing" in her chest in rhythm with the audible swish of the turbine blades. She interpreted this as her "heart synchronized to the rhythm of the blades," but there is no information (such as a pulse rate from the wrist at the same time) to determine whether this was true or not, or whether she detected a separate type of pulsation. Mrs. E could make these sensations go away by getting up and moving around, but they started again when she lay back down.

- Mr. D (D1, age 64) felt pulsations when he lay down in bed. In addition, "When the turbines get into a particular position (facing me), I get real nervous, almost like tremors going through your body... it's more like a vibration from outside... your whole body feels it, as if something was vibrating me, like sitting in a vibrating chair but my body's not moving." This occurs day or night, but not if the turbines are facing "off to the side."

- Mr. C (C1, age 45) felt pulsations in his chest that would induce him to hold his breath, fight the sensation in his chest, and not breathe "naturally." Chest pulsations interrupted his sleep and ability to read. He also described a sensation of "energy coming within me... like being cooked alive in a microwave."

- Mrs. B (B2, age 53) described her breath being "short every once in a while, like [while] falling asleep, my breathing wanted to catch up with something."

- Mr. B (B1, age 55) had two episodes of feeling weight on his chest while lying down, which resolved when he stood up. Other than this, he experienced the invasive quality of the noise in his head and ears: "That stuff [turbine noise] doesn't get out of your head, it gets in there and just sits there—it's horrible."

Agitation, anxiety, alarm, irritability, nausea, tachycardia, and sleep disturbance are associated with internal vibration or pulsation:

- Dr. J's (J1, age 49) "jittery" feeling includes being "real anxious," irritable, and "no fun to be around." He interrupts outdoor and family activities to sequester himself in his well-insulated house. When the turbine blades are spinning fast and he detects certain types of noise and vibration as he arrives home from work, he gets queasy and loses his appetite. He awakens from sleep with the "jittery" feeling and tachycardia, and may need to go downstairs to a cot in the 55-degree root cellar (the only place on his property where he cannot hear or feel the turbines) to be able to fall back to sleep. He often takes deep breaths or sighs when in the "jittery" state.

- Mrs. I (I2, age 52) describes episodic "queasiness and nausea" with loss of appetite, "trembling in arms, legs, fingers," "strong mental and physical agitation," and frequent unexpected crying. On noisy nights she awakens after four hours of sleep, weeping in the night. "When I wake up, [there is] more a feeling of pressure and tightness in my chest; it makes me panic and feel afraid." It is "a startling sort of waking up, a feeling there was something and I don't know what it was." Once she awoke thinking there had been an earth tremor (there had not), and twice she has awakened with tachycardia, the "feeling your heart is beating very fast and very loud, so I can feel the blood pumping." Feelings of panic keep her from going back to sleep.

- Mrs. H (H2, age 57) awakens 5–6 times per night with a feeling of fear and a compulsion to check the house. She describes it as a "very disturbed sort of waking up, you jolt awake, like someone has broken a pane of glass to get into the house. You know what it is but you've got to check it—go open the front door—it's horrific." She finds it hard to fall back to sleep and describes herself as irritable and angry, shouting more at her family members.

- Mr. G (G1, age 35) described the noise outside his home and the noise that awakened him at night as "stressful."

- Mrs. G (G2, age 32) was, during exposure, irritable, angry, and worried about the future and her children. She awoke often at night because her children woke up, when she cared for their fears, mentioning none of her own.

- Mrs. F (F2, age 51) described a "feeling of unease all the time." At night she startles awake with heart pounding, a feeling of fear, and a compulsion to check the house. The feeling of alarm keeps her from being able to go back to sleep.

- Mrs. E (E2, age 56) did not express anxiety or fear, but she awakened repeatedly at night and was unable to get back to sleep on nights when the turbines were facing the house.
- Mr. D (D1, age 64) described how he has to "calm down" from the "tremor." If outside, "I come in, sit down in my chair and try to calm myself down. After an episode like that, I'm real tired." Mood has worsened with increased anger, frustration, and aggression. Tachycardia accompanies the "tremor" at times: "My heart feels like it's starting to race like crazy and I have these tremors going through my body." Mr. D pants or hyperventilates when the tremor and tachycardia occur, and consciously slows his breathing when calming down.
- Mr. C (C1, age 45) was unable to rest, relax, or recuperate in his home, where his body was "always in a state of defense." He had to drive away in his car to rest.
- Mrs. B (B2, age 53) became "upset and in a turmoil" when her symptoms worsened, leaving her house and tasks repeatedly to get relief.
- Mr. B (B1, age 55) described stress, "lots, pretty near more'n I could take, it just burnt me, the noise and run-around." He was prescribed an anxiolytic, and spent more time at the shore in his fishing boat for symptom relief.

The internal quivering, vibration, or pulsation and the associated complex of agitation, anxiety, alarm, irritability, tachycardia, nausea, and sleep disturbance together make up what I refer to as *Visceral Vibratory Vestibular Disturbance* (VVVD). Fourteen adult subjects (six men age 35–64 and eight women age 32–75) had VVVD during exposure, including the eleven quoted above and Mr. F (F1, age 42), Mrs. F Senior (F4, age 75), and Mrs. C (C2, age 42). Mr. I (I1, age 59) had partial symptoms, with an urge to escape, noise-induced nausea, and sleep disturbance, but no feeling of internal movement. VVVD resolves immediately upon leaving the vicinity of the turbines, when the turbines are still and silent, and under favorable weather conditions at each locality.

Because VVVD is in part a panic attack, accompanied by other physical and mental symptoms, I examined the relationships among VVVD and panic disorder, other mental health diagnoses, and other risk factors. The sample for this analysis was 21 adults ages 22 and above (since the study had no participants age 22–29, this is the same for this study as starting with the age group of the youngest symptomatic subjects, who were 32).

No study subjects had pre-existing panic disorder or previous isolated episodes of panic, so there was no correlation between pre-existing panic and VVVD. Seven subjects had mental health disorders either at the time turbines started up near their homes (two subjects) or in the past (five subjects), including depression, anxiety, post-traumatic stress disorder (PTSD), and bipolar disorder. There was no correlation between current or past mental health disorder and VVVD ($\chi^2 = 0.429$, $p = 0.513$). There was, however, a highly significant correlation between VVVD and motion sensitivity ($\chi^2 = 7.88$, $p = 0.005$).

There was also a moderately significant correlation between VVVD and headaches during exposure ($\chi^2 = 4.95$, $p = 0.026$). There was no correlation between VVVD and dizziness or tinnitus during exposure, or between VVVD and pre-existing migraine, tinnitus, or hearing loss.

Concentration and memory. Twenty of the 34 subjects age 4 and up (eleven males age 6–64 and nine females aged 5–56) had salient problems with concentration or memory during exposure to wind turbines, compared to pre- and/or post-exposure. This is a conservative count, including only subjects whose accounts included specific information on decline in school and homework performance (for children and teens) or details on loss of function for adults. Eight other subjects had some disturbance to concentration and memory, but symptoms were milder or the descriptions more vague (in their own or parents' accounts). Five other subjects, all older adults, noted no change compared to pre-existing memory problems. This leaves only one subject, a 19-year-old woman home from college and minimally exposed (B3), who did not have baseline deficits and was unaffected.

Pre-exposure cognitive, educational, and work accomplishments, specific difficulties related to concentration and memory during exposure, and degree and timing of post-exposure recovery are documented in the CASE HISTORIES for each individual, under "Cognition." Difficulties are often striking compared to the subject's usual state of functioning:

- Mr. A (A1, age 32), a professional fisherman with his own boat, who had an isolated difficulty with memory for names and faces prior to exposure, became routinely unable to remember what he meant to get when he arrived at a store, unless he had written it down.
- Mrs. B (B2, age 53), a homemaker, got confused when she went to town for errands unless she had written down what she was going to do, and had to return home to get her list. When interviewed six weeks after moving, she reported that she had improved to being able to manage three things to do without a list.
- Mr. C (C1, age 45) had to put reading aside because he could not concentrate whenever he felt pulsations.

- Mrs. C (C2, age 42), a very organized mother of six who was "ready a month in advance for birthday parties" prior to exposure, became disorganized and had difficulty tracking multiple tasks at once, including while cooking, repeatedly boiling the water away from pots on the stove. She remarked, "I thought I was half losing my mind."
- Mr. D (D1, age 64), a disabled, retired industrial engineer, noticed progressive slowing of memory recall speed and more difficulty remembering what he had read.
- Mrs. E (E2, age 56), a retired teacher active in community affairs, could not spell, write emails, or keep her train of thought on the telephone when the turbine blades were turned towards the house, but was able to do these things when the blades were not facing the house.
- Mrs. F (F2, age 51), a nurse, child development specialist, midwife, and master's level health administrator, could not follow recipes, the plots of TV shows, or furniture assembly instructions during exposure.
- Mrs. G (G2, age 32), a well-organized mother of four, was forgetful, had to write everything down, could not concentrate, and could not get organized. She forgot a child's hearing test appointment. She did not have memory or concentration problems during a previous depression at age 18, and described her experience as "different this time."
- Mr. I (I1, age 59), a professional gardener, could not concentrate on his outdoor gardening and building tasks if the turbines were noisy, saying "after half an hour you have to leave, escape, close the door."
- Dr. J (J1, page 49), a physician, noticed marked concentration problems when he sat down to pay bills in a small home office with a window towards the turbines.

Decline in school performance compared to pre-exposure, or marked improvement in school performance after moving away from turbines, was noted for 7 of the 10 study children and teens attending school (age 5–17; C7, F3, G3, G4, H3, J3, J4). For example:

- A 17-year-old girl (F3), a diligent student, was not concerned about the turbines and thought her parents were overdoing their concern until she unexpectedly did worse on national exams than the previous year, surprising her school, family, and self. At this point she began accompanying her parents to their sleeping house.
- A 9-year-old boy (C7), whose schoolwork was satisfactory without need for extra help prior to exposure, failed tests, lost his math skills, and forgot his math facts. He could not maintain his train of thought during homework, losing track of where he was if he looked up from a problem.
- A 6-year-old boy (G3), described as an extremely focused child and advanced in reading prior to exposure, did not like to read during exposure. Two months post-exposure, now age 7, he would sit down to read on his own for an hour at a time, reading "quite a thick book" for his age.
- His 5-year-old sister (G4) had a short attention span prior to exposure. Her hearing loss due to bilateral chronic serous otitis media was thought to be interfering with schoolwork during exposure, and she repeatedly had tantrums over schoolwork at home during the exposure period. Two months after moving, despite no change in her ears (on a waiting list for pressure equalization tubes), she was more patient and could work longer on homework. Her mother noted that her "schoolwork has improved massively."
- An 8-year-old boy (H3) had an excellent memory and did well in reading, spelling, and math prior to exposure. During exposure he became resistant to doing homework, with tantrums, and

his teacher told him he was not concentrating and needed to go to bed earlier.

In comparing the 20 subjects with salient concentration or memory changes to the 14 who had no change from baseline or vague/minimal difficulties, there are significant relationships with 1) baseline cognition, in that those without memory or concentration deficits at baseline are more likely to notice such deficits during exposure ($\chi^2 = 4.86$, $p = 0.027$), and 2) fatigue or loss of energy or enjoyment for usual activities during exposure ($\chi^2 = 5.61$, $p = 0.018$). There is no significant relationship between salient concentration or memory changes and pre-existing psychiatric diagnoses, migraine, motion sensitivity, or noise exposure, or between salient concentration or memory changes and headache, tinnitus, VVVD, or irritability during exposure.

In addition to the statistical association between fatigue and concentration disturbance, a number of subjects directly attributed their concentration problems to their sleep deprivation or disturbance. Several aspects of the data, however, suggest that additional factors may be involved.

First, one subject, Mrs. E (E2, age 56), could not do certain mental tasks requiring concentration when the turbines were turned towards her house, but could do them when the turbines were not turned towards the house. Mr. C (C1, age 45), Mr. I (I1, age 59), and Dr. J (J1, age 49) also had concentration problems closely linked in time and space to direct exposure to turbine noise.

Second, some of the problems described by subjects, such as Mrs. F (F2, age 51) and the members of families A and B, are more extreme than I expect from sleep deprivation. The degree of thinking dysfunction involved in not being able to follow a recipe or assemble a piece of furniture, in a woman both highly educated and involved in several practical professions (nursing and farming), does not match my expectation of sleep deprivation from the experience, for example, of both younger and older physicians, who often function under sleep deprivation.

Third, some subjects had concentration problems without obvious sleep problems. All four members of family J had concentration problems, but only Dr. J (J1, age 49) was sleep deprived. Mrs. J (J2, age 47) fell asleep easily and usually went back to sleep if awakened, but still had problems with memory and focus in her home activities that she had noticed and attempted to treat. Their 13-year-old son (J3) needed white noise or music to drown out turbine noise to fall asleep, but went to sleep promptly, slept through the night, and did not complain in the morning of being tired or having slept poorly. His school performance and his level of distractibility at home, however, were both markedly different than at baseline. The younger son, age 8 (J4), continued to sleep well, but still had a surprising decline in school performance, though milder and of shorter duration than his brother's.

Fourth, the problems with concentration and memory resolve on a different schedule from the turbine-related sleep problems. Sleep problems resolve immediately except when accompanied by persistent depression (C1, F1). Problems with concentration and memory frequently took longer to improve, even in the absence of depression. To study resolution, we need to look at subjects who have moved away from their exposed homes or spent a prolonged period away that included work (families A, B, C, E, F, and G, and Mrs. I), since vacations do not provide the same challenges to concentration and memory. Of these 23 subjects over age 4, 13 had salient difficulties with concentration or memory:

- Mr. A (A1, age 32) rated his memory as 85% at baseline, 2% during exposure, and 10% six weeks after moving away.

- Mr. and Mrs. B (B1, B2, age 55 and 53) said their memories had partially recovered six weeks after moving.
- Mr. C (C1, now age 47), with continuing depression and ongoing exposure for house maintenance, noted 25 months after moving how bad his memory seemed.
- Mrs. C (C2, now age 44) felt she had recovered her memory and concentration 18 months after moving, despite ongoing stress from crowded living arrangements. Her affected son (now age 11, C7) had not completely recovered his school performance.
- Mrs. E (age 52) recovered immediately. She only experienced problems during exposure when the turbines were turned in a particular direction.
- Mr. and Mrs. F (F1, F2, ages 42 and 51) had moved away but still worked at their turbine-exposed home and farm during the day. Three months after they moved, both thought their concentration had improved, but not to baseline. Mr. F, with ongoing depression, did not perceive any memory recovery. I do not have information about their daughter's (F3, age 17) exam performance after moving.
- Mrs. G (G2, age 32) rated her memory as 10/10 at baseline, 2/10 during exposure, and 5/10 two months after moving away, at which point her depression was mostly resolved. Mrs. G's 5-year-old and 6-year-old children (G3, G4) showed marked improvements in concentration by two months after moving.

Only three subjects were clearly depressed during or after exposure. Mrs. G (G2, age 32) was becoming depressed at the time of the first (during exposure) interview. She remarked on the difference in her cognitive functioning between her current experience and a previous episode of depression at age 18, when she had no problem with her memory or concentration. Two other subjects, Mr. C (C1, age 45) and Mr. F (F1, age 42), developed depression after they had to abandon their homes, which was associated with prolonged memory difficulties. Both also had ongoing exposure.

Irritability and anger. Twenty-eight subjects (15 male age 2–64 and 13 female age 2–64) perceived themselves or were noted by parents to be more angry, irritable, easily frustrated, impatient, rude, defiant, or prone to outbursts or tantrums than at baseline. The adults were uniformly apologetic about their own irritability, and several described how careful they were to avoid acting irritable in their households. Four children (three boys age 8–9 and a girl age 5; C7, G3, H3, G4) were markedly frustrated over homework. The young children of family G quarreled and had tantrums incessantly, and the six children/young adults in family C became angry, prickly, moody, defiant, or prone to fights at school. In families with children, the breakdown in children's behavior, social coping skills, and school performance was one of the strongest elements propelling them to move.

Fatigue and motivation. Twenty-one subjects felt or acted tired, and 24 had problems with motivation for usual, necessary, or formerly enjoyable activities (27 combined, 14 male age 2–64 and 13 female age 2–75). Like concentration and memory, these symptoms undoubtedly have a relationship with sleep deprivation, but certain subjects described leaden feelings around turbines that resolved as soon as they left the vicinity, such as Mr. A (A1, age 32), who said, "You feel different up there: draggy, worn out before you even start anything.... It was a chore to walk across the yard." After driving an hour away to visit a family member, "I felt better all over, like you could do a cart wheel," and he felt well after moving.

When away from their turbine-exposed homes, most subjects recovered their baseline positive mood states, energy, and motivation immediately. Six adult subjects did not. These were Mr. B (B1, age 55), Mr. and Mrs. C (C1, C2, age 45 and 42), Mr. and

Mrs. F (F1, F2, age 42 and 51), and Mrs. G (G2, age 32). By their own accounts, three (Mr. C, Mr. F, and Mrs. G) had unresolved or resolving depression. All but Mrs. G had ongoing anxiety and anger over abandoning their homes and their unresolved life situations.

Other symptom clusters and isolated problems
These symptoms and problems occurred in fewer subjects and typically require more than a medical history to diagnose. Several are exacerbations of pre-existing conditions with obvious connections to situations of high stress or stress hormone (epinephrine, cortisol) output (cardiac arrhythmias, hypertension, irritable bowel, gastroesophageal reflux, glucose instability). One is an extension of a core symptom (unusual migraine aura). Others may indicate different kinds of direct effects of noise on body tissues, as in the vibroacoustic disease model of noise effects (respiratory infections, asthma, clotting abnormalities),[31] or other types of secondary effects (asthma).[32]

Respiratory infection/inflammation cluster. Seven subjects had unusual or prolonged lower respiratory infections during exposure (A2, B1, C2, E2, F1, F3, F4), and two of these also had prolonged asthma exacerbations (F1, F3). These two, however, were also taking a lot of paracetamol (acetaminophen) for their turbine-associated headaches. Four subjects had unusually severe or prolonged middle ear problems (C7, F2, G3, G4).

---

[31] Castelo Branco and Alves-Pereira 2004.

[32] Beasley R, Clayton T, Crane J, von Mutius E, Lai CK, Montefort S, Stewart A; ISAAC Phase Three Study Group. 2008. Association between paracetamol use in infancy and childhood, and the risk of asthma, rhinoconjunctivitis, and eczema in children aged 6–7 years: analysis from Phase Three of the ISAAC programme. Lancet 372(9643): 1039–48.

Cardiovascular cluster. Two subjects had exacerbations of preexisting dysrhythmias (F1, J2). Two women had hypertension that increased during and after the exposure period, requiring medication after the end of exposure. Both still had considerable stress related to moving out and not being able to establish another regular home, and depressed husbands (C2, F2).

Gastrointestinal cluster. Four subjects had exacerbations of preexisting gastroesophageal reflux (GER), ulcer, or irritable bowel, two with irritable bowel and upper gastrointestinal symptoms at the same time (D1, F1, F2, J2).

Arthralgia/myalgia cluster. One healthy 32-year-old woman (G2) noted pain in one elbow while in her exposed house. It resolved when she went away for vacations with her family, and recurred when she returned. It resolved quickly when the family moved away, even though she did lots of lifting during the move. A 57-year-old woman (H2) with lupus arthritis and fibromyalgia at baseline experienced painful exacerbations whenever she returned home, with return to baseline when away. A 56-year-old woman (E2) with fibromyalgia at baseline had exacerbations which resolved during times away from her exposed home and after moving.

Diabetes control. A 56-year-old man with Type II diabetes (E1), stable on oral medications and insulin before exposure, had marked glucose instability accompanied by visual blurring, retinal changes, and polyuria during exposure.

Anticoagulation. A 75-year-old woman with atrial fibrillation (F4) had stable INR values on 2–4 mcg warfarin daily for 10 years. By 16 months of exposure, her warfarin dose had been increased to 8–9 mcg daily in response to decreasing INR values.

Ocular cluster. Three subjects exposed to the same turbines (two men age 32–55 and one woman age 53; A1, B1, B2) had ocular pain, pressure, and/or burning synchronously with headache and tinnitus. Mr. D (D1, age 64) had a painless retinal stroke, losing half the vision in his left eye. Mr. D had a normal CT scan of the brain and was examined by an ophthalmologist.

Complex migraine phenomena. A 19-year-old fisherman (C4) with migraine at baseline had complex visual symptoms with flashes in square patterns in one eye at a time (scintillating scotoma), evolving to blurring and visual loss for 30 seconds to 2 minutes, also in one eye at a time (amaurosis fugax), right more than left, repetitively during the last month of his 15–21 month exposure until 8–12 months after exposure ended, with a decrease in frequency by 7 months after moving out. These events happened at any time of day and rarely overlapped with headaches or tinnitus. He had normal ophthalmologic exams, normal MRI and MRA scans of the brain and associated arteries, and a normal evaluation for clotting abnormalities and vasculitis. The events resolved completely with normal vision. The same man experienced repetitive complex basilar migraines with aura after the first few months of his 15–21 month turbine exposure, involving daily bilateral paresis and paresthesias of his legs and occasional headache, tinnitus, and light-headedness. The leg symptoms resolved on the same schedule as the eye symptoms, though headaches and nausea continue to be triggered regularly by seasickness.

Discussion

The core symptoms of Wind Turbine Syndrome are sleep disturbance, headache, tinnitus, other ear and hearing sensations, disturbances to balance and equilibrium, nausea, anxiety, irritability, energy loss, motivation loss, disturbances to memory and concentration, and *Visceral Vibratory Vestibular Disturbance*

(VVVD). Core symptoms are defined as common and widely described by study participants, closely linked in time and space to turbine exposure, and amenable to diagnosis by medical history. The latter was a particular requirement of this study. The subjects of this study had other types of health problems during exposure, discussed in "Other symptom clusters and isolated problems," but different types of study will be needed to find out if there is a link between these problems and wind turbine exposure.

The most distinctive feature of Wind Turbine Syndrome is the group of symptoms I call *Visceral Vibratory Vestibular Disturbance*. The adults who experience this describe a feeling of internal pulsation, quivering, or jitteriness, accompanied by nervousness, anxiety, fear, a compulsion to flee or check the environment for safety, nausea, chest tightness, and tachycardia. The symptoms arise day or night, interrupting daytime activities and concentration, and interrupting sleep. Wakefulness is prolonged after this type of awakening. Subjects observe that their symptoms occur in association with specific types of turbine function: the turbines turned directly towards or away from them, running particularly fast, or making certain types of noise. The symptoms create aversive reactions to bedroom and house. Subjects tend to be irritable and frustrated, especially over the loss of their ability to rest and be revitalized at home. Subjects with VVVD are also prone to queasiness and loss of appetite even when the full set of symptoms is not present.

There is no statistical association in this study between VVVD and pre-existing panic episodes (which occurred in none of the subjects) or other mental health disorders, such as depression, anxiety, bipolar disorder, or post-traumatic stress disorder. There is a highly significant association between VVVD and pre-existing motion sensitivity ($p = 0.005$).

Headaches more frequent or severe than at baseline occurred in all migraineurs in the study, and all children with headaches in the study were migraineurs or the children of migraineurs. Non-migrainous adults also got severe headaches around turbines, and indeed about half the people with headache worse than baseline (9 out of 19) were adults without history of migraine. Pre-exposure migraine is a significant risk factor for more severe or frequent headaches during turbine exposure ($p = 0.004$), but does not account for all the cases of headache.

Tinnitus occurred as a migraine aura in three subjects, but statistically in the study group tinnitus was not significantly associated with pre-existing migraine disorder, but rather with sensations of ear popping, pressure, or pain during exposure ($p = 0.008$), previous industrial noise exposure ($p = 0.013$), past history of tinnitus ($p = 0.017$), baseline permanent hearing impairment ($p = 0.040$), and (weakly) with dizziness/disequilibrium during exposure ($p = 0.058$). Like the other core symptoms, tinnitus resolved or returned to baseline when subjects were away from turbines. Previous noise exposure, past tinnitus, and baseline hearing impairment all suggest prior damage to the cochlea as a risk factor. The co-occurring symptoms of ear popping, pressure, and pain during exposure suggest that tinnitus may be caused near turbines by transient alterations in inner-ear fluid pressures (perilymph or endolymph). The weak correlation between tinnitus and dizziness/disequilibrium suggests that the proposed pressure shift may concurrently affect vestibular organ function.

Visceral Vibratory Vestibular Disturbance (VVVD)
The work of Mittelstaedt on visceral detectors of gravity,[33,34] and

---

[33] Mittelstaedt H. 1996. Somatic graviception. Biol Psychol 42(1–2): 53–74.

[34] Mittelstaedt H. 1999. The role of the otoliths in perception of the vertical and in path integration. Ann N Y Acad Sci 871: 334–44.

Balaban and others on balance-anxiety linkages,[35–39] opens a window on the VVVD symptom set. Balaban, a neuroscientist, has localized and described the neural connections among the vestibular organs of the inner ear, brain nuclei involved with balance processing, autonomic and somatic sensory inflow and outflow, the fear and anxiety associated with vertigo or a sudden feeling of postural instability, and aversive learning.[40] These form a coordinated, neurologically integrated system based in the parabrachial nucleus of the brainstem and an associated neural network.[41,42] Several aspects of this system need to be considered here.

First, there appear to be not three but four body systems for regulating balance, upright posture, and the sense of position and motion in space.[43,44] The first three systems are the eyes, the semicircular canals and otolith organs of the inner ear (vestibular organs), and somatic input from skin, skeletal muscles, tendons,

---

[35] Balaban CD, Yates BJ. 2004. The vestibuloautonomic interactions: a teleologic perspective. Chapter 7 in *The Vestibular System*, ed. Highstein SM, Fay RR, Popper AN, pp. 286–342. Springer-Verlag, New York.

[36] Balaban CD. 2002. Neural substrates linking balance control and anxiety. Physiology and Behavior 77: 469–75.

[37] Furman JM, Balaban CD, Jacob RG. 2001. Interface between vestibular dysfunction and anxiety: more than just psychogenicity. Otol Neurotol 22(3): 426–27.

[38] Balaban CD. 2004. Projections from the parabrachial nucleus to the vestibular nuclei: potential substrates for autonomic and limbic influences on vestibular responses. Brain Res 996: 126–37.

[39] Halberstadt A, Balaban CD. 2003. Organization of projections from the raphe nuclei to the vestibular nuclei in rats. Neuroscience 120(2): 573–94.

[40] Balaban and Yates 2004.

[41] Balaban CD, Thayer JF. 2001. Neurological bases for balance-anxiety links. J Anx Disord 15: 53–79.

[42] Balaban 2002.

[43] Mittelstaedt 1996.

[44] Mittelstaedt 1999.

and joints (somatosensory system). The fourth system is visceral detection of gravity, upright position, and acceleration (meaning change in speed or direction of movement) by *visceral graviceptors*. These include stretch receptors in mesenteries or other connective tissue supporting organs or great vessels, and integrated systems of pressure detection in vessels and organs.[45] Such receptors have been localized to the kidneys and to the great vessels or their supporting structures in the mediastinum.[46] Mittelstaedt shows (by clever calculation and experimentation with people positioned in various ways on spinning centrifuge tables in the dark) that the visceral graviceptors control about 60% of our perception of position relative to gravity (meaning our sense of whether we are vertical or horizontal, or somewhere in between), compared to a 40% contribution made by the otolith organs.[47] Von Gierke (an older dean of vibration studies for the US space program) considers an inter-modality sensory conflict related to phase differences between the abdominal visceral graviceptors and the otolith organs to be a possible cause of motion sickness.[48]

The second critical element is central processing: how sensory information about motion and position is integrated by the brain, what other brain centers are activated, and what kinds of signals the brain then sends back to the body. Balaban and colleagues describe how the parabrachial nucleus network receives motion and position information from visual, vestibular (inner ear), somatosensory, and visceral sensory input, and is linked to brain

---

[45] Balaban and Yates 2004.

[46] Vaitl D, Mittelstaedt H, Baisch F. 2002. Shifts in blood volume alter the perception of posture: further evidence for somatic graviception. Int J Psychophysiol 44(1): 1–11.

[47] Mittelstaedt 1999.

[48] von Gierke HE, Parker DE. 1994. Differences in otolith and abdominal viscera graviceptor dynamics: implications for motion sickness and perceived body position. Aviat Space Environ Med 65(8): 747–51.

centers and circuits that mediate anxiety and fear, including the amygdala (a key mediator of fear reactions) and serotonin and norepinephrine-bearing neurons radiating from the midbrain.[49–51] Meaning that our sense of balance and stability in space is closely connected—neurologically—to fear and anxiety.

Balaban illustrates with a story. He asks the reader to visualize waiting in traffic on a hill for a light to turn. Out of the corner of your eye you see the truck next to you starting to inch forward, and you jam your foot on the brake, since your sensory system has told you that you are starting to slip backwards. There's a bit of panic in that moment, quickly settled as you realize you are indeed stable in space and not moving. The story illustrates how a sensation of unexpected movement elicits alerting and fear. When the sense of movement is ongoing and cannot be integrated with the evidence of the other senses, as happens in vertigo, there is a more prolonged fear reaction. In fact, as Balaban shows, the association of fear with vertigo has been known since ancient times.[52]

The third critical element is integrated neurologic outflow to the body from the parabrachial nucleus network to both the somatic (conscious, voluntary) and visceral (autonomic) effector systems. The somatic musculature is responsible for that fast foot on the brake, for righting movements of limbs, torso, and neck, and for breathing motions of the diaphragm and chest wall. The autonomic system is responsible for blood flow, heart rate, blood pressure, sweating, nausea, and other automatic, non-conscious modifications to visceral functioning. In a fear response, there is integrated outflow to these two systems—the somatic and visceral/

---

[49] Balaban and Thayer 2001.
[50] Balaban 2002.
[51] Halberstadt and Balaban 2003.
[52] Balaban and Thayer 2001.

autonomic. Experimental work with animals shows that vestibular signaling has profound effects on autonomic regulation of body temperature, heart rate, vascular resistance, and circadian rhythms of activity and hormone secretion.[53,54] These effects extend to humans. Vestibular stimulation by passive linear acceleration causes blood pressure and heart rate increases, with diminished responses in people with reduced vestibular function.[55]

The parabrachial nucleus network is also involved in aversive learning,[56] an experience in which nausea, if present, plays a dominant role.[57]

In VVVD, subjects detect unusual types of movement (pulsation, internal vibration, internal quivering) or other sensations (pressure, a sense of fighting something to breathe, pins and needles) in the chest or in the coordinated chest-abdominal internal space. The chest and abdomen are separated and unified by the diaphragm, which, as a striated somatic muscle, has fine-grained sensitivity to motion and stretch. The diaphragm sends signals to the brain which are specific and localizable in time and space, as opposed to visceral receptors, which send signals that are vague, like discomfort, malaise, fullness, or nausea. The diaphragm is tightly

---

[53] Murakami DM, Erkman L, Hermanson O, Rosenfeld MG, Fuller CA. 2002. Evidence for vestibular regulation of autonomic functions in a mouse genetic model. Proc Natl Acad Sci USA 99(26): 17078–82.

[54] Wilson TD, Cotter LA, Draper JA, Misra SP, Rice CD, Cass SP, Yates BJ. 2006. Vestibular inputs elicit patterned changes in limb blood flow in conscious cats. J Physiol 575(2): 671–84.

[55] Yates BJ, Aoki M, Burchill P, Bronstein AM. 1999. Cardiovascular responses elicited by linear acceleration in humans. Exp Brain Res 125: 476–84.

[56] Balaban and Thayer 2001.

[57] Garcia J, Ervin FR. 1968. Gustatory-visceral and telereceptor-cutaneous conditioning: adaptation in internal and external milieus. Commun Behav Biol 1: 389–415.

bound to one of the largest abdominal organs, the liver, and they move as a unit during breathing.

The chest, via the mouth, nose, trachea, smaller airways, and air sacs of the lungs, is open to the air. Pressure fluctuations in the air (sound waves) have free access to this airspace within the body when we breathe. Pressure fluctuations in the air also have access to the ear, which is designed to funnel them to the tympanic membrane, which concentrates their energy and transmits it to the inner ear. The ear and the chest are different size spaces with walls of different mobility and elasticity. Hence they respond differently to air pressure fluctuations (sound waves) of different sizes.

Studies of whole-body vibration focus on the easily mobile diaphragm and coupled abdominal organs. Being mobile, with the air of the lungs on one side and the soft abdominal wall on the other, this thoraco-abdominal system is easily set in motion by lower energy (amplitude) vibrations than are required to perturb other parts of the body.[58] Each part of the body has its own resonance frequency with regard to vibration. When an object is vibrated at its resonance frequency, the vibration is amplified. The resonant frequency of the thoraco-abdominal system, as it moves vertically towards and away from the lungs, lies between 4 and 8 Hz for adult humans.[59] Vibrations between 4 and 6 Hz set up resonances in the trunk with amplification up to 200%.[60] Related chest and abdominal effects are found in the same frequency range. Vibrations in the 4–8 Hz range influence breathing movements, 5–7 Hz can cause chest pains, 4–10 Hz abdominal pains, and 4–9

---

[58] Coermann RR, Ziegenruecker GH, Wittwer AL, von Gierke HE. 1960. The passive dynamic mechanical properties of the human thorax-abdominal system and of the whole body system. Aerosp Med 31(6): 443–55.

[59] von Gierke and Parker 1994.

[60] Hedge 2007.

Hz a general feeling of discomfort.[61] In small children under 40 pounds, the vertical resonance or power absorption peaks at 7.5 Hz, as opposed to 4–5 Hz for adults.[62]

Low frequency noise can cause the human body to vibrate, as quantified by researchers in Japan.[63] The degree to which the body surface is induced to vibrate by low frequency noise is correlated with subjective unpleasantness (a sensation suggesting visceral as well as surface/somatic stimulation by the noise).[64]

With this background, I propose the following mechanism for VVVD. Air pressure fluctuations in the range of 4–8 Hz, which may be harmonics of the turbine blade-passing frequency, may resonate (amplify) in the chest and be felt as vibrations or quivering of the diaphragm with its attached abdominal organ mass (liver). Slower air pressure fluctuations, which could be the blade-passing frequencies themselves or a low harmonic (1–2 Hz), would be felt as pulsations, as opposed to the faster vibrations or quivering. (The vibrations or pressure fluctuations may also be occurring at different frequencies, without this particular resonance amplification.) The pressure fluctuations in the chest could disturb visceral receptors, such as large vessel or pulmonary baroreceptors or mediastinal stretch receptors which function as visceral graviceptors. These aberrant signals from the visceral graviceptors, not concordant with signals from the other parts of the motion-detecting system, have the potential to activate

---

[61] Rasmussen 1982.

[62] Giacomin J. 2005. Absorbed power of small children. Clin Biomech 20(4): 372–80.

[63] Takahashi Y, Yonekawa Y, Kanada K, Maeda S. 1999. A pilot study on the human body vibration induced by low-frequency noise. Ind Health 37: 28–35.

[64] Takahashi Y, Kanada K, Yonekawa Y, Harada N. 2005. A study on the relationship between subjective unpleasantness and body surface vibrations induced by high-level low-frequency pure tones. Ind Health 43: 580–87, p. 580.

the integrated neural networks that link motion detection with somatic and autonomic outflow, emotional fear responses, and aversive learning. The people who are susceptible to responding in this way are those who in the past have become nauseated in response to other vertically oriented, anomalous environmental movements (seasickness or carsickness). Thus panic episodes with autonomic symptoms such as tachycardia and nausea arise during wakefulness or sleep in people with pre-existing motion sensitivity but without prior history of panic, anxiety, or other mental health disorders. Repeated triggering of these symptoms creates aversive learning, wherein the person begins to feel horror and dread of things associated with the physical sensations, such as his bedroom or house where he previously found comfort and regeneration.

VVVD was identified in the study in 14 out of 21 adult subjects. The behavior and experiences of other subjects, especially children, could be interpreted as partial manifestations of the same problem. For example, the two toddlers in the study, both age 2½ (A3, G5), had night terrors. They awoke screaming multiple times per night, and were inconsolable and difficult to get back to sleep. The little girl (G5) would fight her mother, grabbing onto the posts of the bunk bed, to avoid going back into her own bed after awakening in this state. This shows clear parallels with the fear responses, prolonged awake periods, and aversive responses of the adults with VVVD. Both toddlers were agitated and irritable in the daytime, also similar to the adults in the study. Both 5-year-olds in the study, a boy and a girl (C7, G4), also frequently woke up fearful at night.

Perturbing the inner ear
I propose that disrupted stimulation of other channels of the balance system, especially the inner-ear vestibular organs, is also likely to play a role in Wind Turbine Syndrome. Altogether, in subjects with or without VVVD, the Wind Turbine Syndrome core symptoms resemble the symptoms of a balance or vestibular

disorder, meaning malfunctioning of the inner-ear motion-detecting organs (peripheral vestibular dysfunction) or of brain processing of balance-related neural signals (central balance dysfunction). These symptoms may arise near wind turbines due to abnormal stimulation of the classical balance pathways (visual, vestibular, and somatosensory), perhaps in an additive fashion if several pathways are disturbed simultaneously.

A clinical rule of thumb is that two of the three classical balance channels have to be working and producing coherent information (with agreement among channels) for a person to keep his or her balance. (How this clinical rule will incorporate the new fourth channel of balance information is yet to be seen. It may be that the sensory integrative process is actually broader, taking into account the amounts and quality of information coming from each channel, not just whether a channel is active.) The three classical pathways are 1) vision, which includes a) seeing one's orientation relative to objects and the orientation of objects relative to gravity, b) movement of images across the retina, called "retinal slip," and c) parallax or distance detection; 2) somatosensory, which involves stretch signals from muscles, tendons, and joints, and touch sensations from the skin; and 3) signals from the inner-ear vestibular organs.

The vestibular organs are 1) the semicircular canals, which detect angular acceleration during rotation of the head in any of three planes, and 2) the otolith organs (utricle and saccule), which detect gravity, tilt (static or moving), and linear accelerations by virtue of microscopic calcium carbonate crystals (otoconia) positioned in a protein matrix over the sensing hair cells. In the utricle, the patch of hair cells plus otoconia (called the macula) is oriented horizontally and is sensitive to tilts and (in upright people) to the horizontal component of linear accelerations. In the saccule, the macula is vertical, sensitive to tilts and to the vertical component of linear accelerations (including gravity) in upright people. The inner-ear or labyrinthine organs are delicate, membranous, interconnected structures with fluid inside (endolymph) and outside (perilymph), suspended in tiny canals and chambers through solid temporal bone at the base of the skull. The vertically oriented macula of the saccule is firmly bound to temporal bone over its entire area, but the horizontally oriented macula of the utricle has been recently found to be attached to temporal bone only at its anterior end,[65] a property that gives it an additional degree of freedom that may influence its tuning or resonance with regard to vibration.[66] Hair cells, which send neural signals when mechanically perturbed, are also present in specific parts of the semicircular canals and the cochlea, which is the spiral-shaped hearing organ.

In the current study, two subjects (C2, E2) were sensitive to the visual pathway with regard to triggering of symptoms. They developed severe headaches when exposed to the moving shadows of turbine blades. One (C2) had known migraine and was prone to vertigo. The other (E2) had fibromyalgia and a history of two pre-exposure episodes of vertigo. Fibromyalgia, a syndrome of chronic, diffuse pain of central origin,[67] is frequently accompanied by vertigo and dizziness.[68]

---

[65] Uzun-Coruhlu H, Curthoys IS, Jones AS. 2007. Attachment of the utricular and saccular maculae to the temporal bone. Hear Res 233(1–2): 77–85.

[66] Todd NP, Rosengren SM, Colebatch JG. 2009. A utricular origin of frequency tuning to low-frequency vibration in the human vestibular system? Neurosci Lett 451(3): 175–80.

[67] Staud R, Cannon RC, Mauderli AP, Robinson ME, Price DD, Vierck CJ Jr. 2003. Temporal summation of pain from mechanical stimulation of muscle tissue in normal controls and subjects with fibromyalgia syndrome. Pain 102: 87–95.

[68] Rosenhall U, Johansson G, Orndahl G. 1996. Otoneurologic and audiologic findings in fibromyalgia. Scand J Rehabil Med 28(4): 225–32. In this study, 72% of 168 fibromyalgia patients had dizziness or vertigo, most with abnormalities on otoneurologic testing.

Two subjects (C2, J2) noticed vibrations in their lower legs at certain locations on their properties, which opens the possibility of disruption of the somatosensory channel.[69] An audiologist detected vibration in the floor of an affected room in the C family's house, becoming nauseated when he put his forehead against it, an effect he interpreted as stimulation of the vestibular organs by bone conduction.[70]

I suspect that the inner-ear vestibular organs—and the cochlea—are abnormally stimulated in Wind Turbine Syndrome, especially in subjects who have marked ear symptoms such as tinnitus (including the sensation of noise inside the head) and ear pressure, popping, or pain. Families A and B, exposed to the same set of turbines, showed this pattern of symptoms especially strongly. All four adults (A1, A2, B1, B2) also had unsteadiness on their feet without accompanying vertigo or history of migraine, vertigo, prior unsteadiness, or neurologic disease. Unsteady gait, or ataxia, is generally associated with cerebellar dysfunction, but can also indicate otolith dysfunction.[71] (Vestibular nuclei in the brainstem are richly interconnected with the cerebellum.)[72] Other subjects (C2, G1, J1) had vertigo during exposure (C2 also had observed nystagmus), suggesting that disordered signals were reaching the vestibulo-ocular reflex arc from the semicircular canals or otolith organs.

---

[69] Hanes DA, McCollum G. 2006. Cognitive-vestibular interactions: a review of patient difficulties and possible mechanisms. J Vestib Res 16(3): 75–91. Vibration of calf muscles is a method sometimes used in balance studies to simulate somatosensory disturbance, p. 77.

[70] Noise report prepared for family C, May 2006.

[71] Schlindwein P, Mueller M, Bauermann T, Brandt T, Stoeter P, Dieterich M. 2008. Cortical representation of saccular vestibular stimulation: VEMPs in fMRI. Neuroimage 39: 19–31.

[72] Colebatch JG, Halmagyi GM, Skuse NF. 1994. Myogenic potentials generated by a click-evoked vestibulocollic reflex. J Neurol Neurosurg Psychiatry 57(2): 190–97.

In Wind Turbine Syndrome, I hypothesize that low frequency noise or vibration impinges on the delicately mobile labyrinthine organs, but not in a way that stimulates the cochlea to a coherent representation of sound. Instead, the low frequency noise or vibration, I suggest, may stimulate various parts of the labyrinth in a disorganized fashion, experienced as tinnitus from the cochlea, a distorted sense of vertical from the otolith organs, or illusory self-motion from the otolith organs or semicircular canals. The dominant sensory impression may depend on 1) the frequencies and intensities of low frequency noise and vibration coming from the turbines, 2) whether the noise or vibration arrives at the ear through the air and outer/middle ear or is bone-conducted, and 3) the susceptibilities and prior histories of the subjects, such as migraine with its tendency towards vertigo, prior damage to the cochlea, or other conditions or anomalies of the inner ear.[73]

The statistical correlation in the current study between tinnitus and ear popping, pressure, or pain during exposure suggests a refinement to this mechanism: altered fluid pressure relationships in the inner ear may distort cochlear mechanics during exposure and cause tinnitus, and distort utricular and saccular mechanics to create instability or ataxia and other second-order vestibular symptoms.

Low frequency noise, in fact, is known to distort endolymphatic pressure and volume after just short exposures to loud but not

---

[73] For example, dehiscence of the superior semicircular canal, in which alterations in inner-ear pressure relationships due to a "third window" effect (from an abnormal hole in the bone between the superior semicircular canal and the cranial cavity) cause conductive hearing loss, increased sensitivity to bone-conducted sound or vibration, and the tendency to become unbalanced by sounds (Tullio effect). Dislocation of the stapes footplate, labyrinthine fistulas, and endolymphatic hydrops can also underlie the Tullio phenomenon. (See Colebatch JG, Day BL, Bronstein AM, Davies RA, Gresty MA, Luxon LM, Rothwell JC. 1998. Vestibular hypersensitivity to clicks is characteristic of the Tullio phenomenon. J Neurol Neurosurg Psychiatry 65: 670–78.)

damaging low frequency tones.[74] This temporary effect is associated with hyperacusis, a distortion of hearing function in which sounds are perceived as louder.[75] One subject in the current study, G2, had hyperacusis while living near turbines, and another (C2) noticed hyperacusis after her tinnitus resolved, after she moved away from the turbines. Tinnitus may also be associated with increased perilymphatic and intracranial pressure in the presence of an open cochlear aqueduct, which provides a direct channel linking these two fluid spaces.[76]

There is both animal and human precedent for thinking that certain types of environmental noise or vibration may stimulate the otolith organs and cause disturbance to motion and position sense. Vestibular organ structures have been conserved during evolution, meaning they are rather similar in fish, amphibians, and other vertebrate taxa, including humans. All the vertebrates have semicircular canals and otolith organs. Like us, fish use their otolith organs (utricle, saccule, and an extra one, the lagena) to sense linear accelerations and tilt relative to gravity, but these organs in "non-specialist" fish species (such as cod) are also the fishes' auditory organs. The otolith organs in these fish are highly sensitive to nearby perturbations in the water ("near-field sound")[77] with peak sensitivities in the low frequency range between 40 and 120 Hz.[78] Atlantic cod otolith organs are so sensitive to

---

[74] Salt AN. 2004. Acute endolymphatic hydrops generated by exposure of the ear to nontraumatic low-frequency tones. J Assoc Res Otolaryngol 5(2): 203–14.

[75] Salt 2004.

[76] Reid A, Cottingham CA, Marchbanks RJ. 1993. The prevalence of perilymphatic hypertension in subjects with tinnitus: a pilot study. Scand Audiol 22: 61–63.

[77] Sand O, Karlsen HE, Knudsen FR. 2008. Comment on "Silent research vessels are not quiet" [J Acoust Soc Am 2007; 121(4): EL145–50]. J Acoust Soc Am 123(4): 1831–33.

[78] Fay RR, Simmons AM. 1999. The sense of hearing in fishes and amphibians. In *Comparative Hearing: Fish and Amphibians*, ed. Fay RR, Popper AN, pp. 269–317. Springer-Verlag, New York.

infrasound in water (at 0.1 Hz, or one wave every 10 seconds) that the fish may be able to use seismic sounds from the Mid-Atlantic Ridge or the sounds of waves breaking on distant shores, or even more complex mechanisms, to guide them during migration.[79,80] Directional infrasound detection plays a role in predator avoidance behaviors.[81]

In humans, there is a substantial body of experimental evidence showing that both air-conducted sound and bone-conducted sound (vibration) stimulate the otolith organs and cause measurable impacts on vestibular reflexes, independent of their stimulation of the cochlea. Air-borne sound in the form of loud clicks or short tone bursts induces inhibitory neural signals in the sternocleidomastoid muscles in the anterior neck. Called the *vestibular evoked myogenic potential* (VEMP), this is an extremely fast or "short-latency" neural response that is part of the vestibulocollic reflex.[82] Bone-conducted sound or vibration is more efficient than air-conducted clicks or tones at stimulating the otolith organs: both the absolute decibel levels and decibels above hearing threshold needed to produce the VEMP response are lower for bone-conducted sound.[83]

Studies of both the VEMP and—a second measure of vestibular function—the *ocular vestibular evoked myogenic potential* (OVEMP) show that the tuning (best frequency response) for both

---

[79] Sand O, Karlsen HE. 1986. Detection of infrasound by the Atlantic cod. J Exp Biol 125: 197–204.

[80] Sand O, Karlsen HE. 2000. Detection of infrasound and linear acceleration in fishes. Phil Trans R Soc Lond B 355: 1295–98.

[81] Karlsen HE, Piddington RW, Enger PS, Sand O. 2004. Infrasound initiates directional fast-start escape responses in juvenile roach Rutilus rutilus. J Exp Biol 207(Pt 24): 4185–93.

[82] Colebatch et al. 1994.

[83] Welgampola MS, Rosengren SM, Halmagyi GM, Colebatch JG. 2003. Vestibular activation by bone conducted sound. J Neurol Neurosurg Psychiatry 74: 711–18.

VEMP and OVEMP for air-conducted sound lies between 400 and 800 Hz.[84] Whereas with bone-conducted sound (vibration), the best frequency response for both VEMP and OVEMP is at 100 Hz. Modeling of the frequency tuning and other aspects of the response, such as laterality, phase differences, and gain, suggests that the air-conducted peak comes from the rigidly attached saccule, whereas the bone-conducted or vibratory peak derives from the more mobile utricle.[85] A particular type of vestibular hair cell, Type I cells, is thought to be involved in the utricular response and accounts for the marked sensitivity of the OVEMP response to vibration, since these cells typically produce a strong neural vestibular signal in response to a low degree of mechanical disturbance.[86,87]

Most exciting, Todd et al. provide direct experimental evidence that at the 100 Hz tuning peak, the vestibular organs (probably utricle, as above) of normal humans are *much more sensitive than the cochlea* to low frequency bone-conducted sound/vibration.[88] The researchers applied vibration directly to the skin over the bony mastoid prominence behind the subjects' ears, adjusting the power by measuring the tiny whole-head acceleration produced by each vibration force and frequency. They were able to elicit and measure neural signals of the vestibulo-ocular reflex (OVEMP, as above) at vibration intensities 15 dB below the subjects' hearing thresholds. In other words, the amount of vibration/bone-conducted sound was so small that the subjects could not hear it, yet the vestibular parts of their inner ears still responded to the vibration and

---

[84] Todd et al. 2009.

[85] Todd et al. 2009.

[86] Todd et al. 2009.

[87] Curthoys IS, Kim J, McPhedran SK, Camp AJ. 2006. Bone conducted vibration selectively activates irregular primary otolithic vestibular neurons in the guinea pig. Exp Brain Res 175(2): 256–67.

[88] Todd et al. 2008.

transmitted signals into the balance and motion networks in the brain, resulting in specific types of eye muscle activation. Since dB is a base 10 logarithmic measure, *15 dB below* means a signal 0.0316 ($10^{-1.5}$), or about 3%, of the power or amplitude of the signal these normal subjects could hear.

The researchers note that "the very low thresholds we found are remarkable as they suggest that humans possess a frog- or fish-like sensory mechanism which appears to exceed the cochlea for detection of substrate-borne low-frequency vibration and which until now has not been properly recognized."[89] Thus the potential exists, in normal humans, for stimulation of balance signals from the inner ear by low frequency noise and vibration, even when the noise or vibration does not seem especially loud, or even cannot be heard. In the presence of pre-existing inner-ear pathology, thresholds for vestibular stimulation by noise or vibration are even lower than in normal subjects.[90]

Central balance processing

When there is conflict in neurologically normal people among the signals coming from the different balance channels, the brain areas that integrate the information quickly compensate by suppressing or down-weighting information from the anomalous channel[91]— information that does not match what is coming from the other channels. On functional brain scans, vestibular and visual cortical areas show a pattern of inverse activation and deactivation, such

---

[89] Todd et al. 2008, p. 41.

[90] Colebatch et al. 1998. See footnote 73.

[91] Jacob RG, Redfern MS, Furman JM. 2009. Space and motion discomfort and abnormal balance control in patients with anxiety disorders. J Neurol Neurosurg Psychiatry 80(1): 74–78. E-pub 2008 July 24.

that vestibular activation deactivates visual cortex and vice versa.[92,93] In people with vestibular organ damage, long-term compensation promotes reliance on vision ("visual dependence") or on somatosensory input from muscles, tendons, joints, and skin ("surface dependence"). A visually dependent vestibular patient cannot adequately suppress visual input and up-weight vestibular signals because of pre-existing problems with the vestibular channel,[94] leaving the person dependent on visual perception of motion and position even in environments where the visual information is ambiguous. When combined with the sense of fear generated by a feeling of postural instability or uncertainty (as reviewed above), this can create fear of heights.

It can also cause Space and Motion Discomfort,[95] a condition in which situations challenging to motion and position sense create discomfort. These situations include looking up at tall buildings, scanning shelves in a supermarket, closing eyes in the shower, leaning far back in a chair, driving through tunnels, riding in an elevator, riding in the back seat of a car, or reading in the car.[96]

Even without vestibular organ disease, some people have Space and Motion Discomfort due to a central or brain-based difficulty with

---

[92] Brandt T, Bartenstein P, Janek A, Dieterich M. 1998. Reciprocal inhibitory visual-vestibular interaction. Visual motion stimulation deactivates the parieto-insular vestibular cortex. Brain 121(Pt. 9): 1749–58.

[93] Brandt T, Dieterich M. 1999. The vestibular cortex: its locations, functions, and disorders. Ann NY Acad Sci 871: 293–312.

[94] Redfern MS, Yardley L, Bronstein AM. 2001. Visual influences on balance. J Anxiety Disord 15(1–2): 81–94.

[95] Jacob RG, Woody SR, Clark DB, Lilienfeld SO, Hirsch BE, Kucera GD, Furman JM, Durrant JD. 1993. Discomfort with space and motion: a possible marker of vestibular dysfunction assessed by the Situational Characteristics Questionnaire. J Psychopathol Behav Assess 15(4): 299–324.

[96] Jacob et al. 2009. As a rural physician, I might also ask patients about driving past rows of parallel trees, especially with the low winter sun flashing between the trunks, as the rural equivalent of looking at lights on the wall of a tunnel.

the process of integrating balance signals into a coherent, moment-to-moment representation of their motion and orientation in space. Balance testing using posturography shows that such people have difficulty down-weighting anomalous information from either the visual or somatosensory channel, or have a mild, central disorder of balance control with increased postural sway even under non-challenging conditions.[97–99]

Space and Motion Discomfort is common in patients with anxiety disorders,[100,101] migrainous vertigo,[102] and migraine-anxiety related dizziness.[103] Vertigo is especially characteristic of migraine and may at times occur as a migraine aura with or without headache.[104] In one study, dizziness or vertigo was found in 54% of 200 migraine patients, half of whom also had a history of motion sickness, compared with 30% of people with tension-type headaches.[105] In a study of 72 patients with isolated recurrent vertigo, 61% were found to have migraine, compared to 10% in a control group of orthopedic patients.[106] Abnormal balance testing

---

[97] Redfern MS, Furman JM, Jacob RG. 2007. Visually induced postural sway in anxiety disorders. J Anxiety Disord 21(5): 704–16. NIH Public Access Author Manuscript, pp. 1–14.

[98] Jacob et al. 2009.

[99] Furman JM, Balaban CD, Jacob RG, Marcus DA. 2005. Migraine-anxiety related dizziness (MARD): a new disorder? J Neurol Neurosurg Psychiatry 76: 1–8.

[100] Jacob et al. 2009.

[101] Redfern et al. 2007.

[102] Neuhauser H, Leopold M, von Brevern M, Arnold G, Lempert T. 2001. The interactions of migraine, vertigo, and migrainous vertigo. Neurology 56: 436–41.

[103] Furman et al. 2005.

[104] Furman et al. 2005.

[105] Kayan A, Hood JD. 1984. Neuro-otological manifestations of migraine. Brain 107: 1123–42.

[106] Lee H, Sohn SI, Jung DK, Cho YW, Lim JG, Yi SD, Yi HA. 2002. Migraine and isolated recurrent vertigo of unknown cause. Neurol Res 24(7): 663–65.

is seen in patients with migraine but not in those with tension-type headaches.[107] Balance testing shows that both central and vestibular organ balance problems are found in migraine patients, especially in those who experience dizziness or vertigo.[108]

About 50% of migraine sufferers in general have histories of motion sickness, compared to only about 20% in people with tension headaches.[109] Motion sickness is the most common vestibular symptom in migraine. Motion sickness is provoked by excessively moving environments (amusement park rides, boats in rough water, airplanes in turbulence, the back of a school bus) or situations of conflict among visual, vestibular, somatosensory, and visceral signals to the balance system (reading in the car, riding in the back seat, driving in snow, simulators, IMax movies, computer images and games, space travel). The nausea of motion sickness may be accompanied by dizziness, cold sweat, pallor, headache, increased salivation, sleepiness, and apathy or disinclination for physical or mental work, thus sharing many symptoms with migraine.[110] Like migraine, motion sickness is more common in women.[111] Visual migraine aura without headache is increased in adults with a history of childhood motion sickness. Motion sickness is not associated with peripheral vestibular disorders, however, such as benign paroxysmal positional vertigo, Meniere's disease, or vestibular neuritis.[112]

---

[107] Ishizaki K, Mori N, Takeshima T, Fukuhara Y, Ijiri T, Kusumi M, Yasui K, Kowa H, Nakashima K. 2002. Static stabilometry in patients with migraine and tension-type headache during a headache-free period. Psychiatry Clin Neurosci 56(1): 85–90.

[108] Furman et al. 2005.

[109] Marcus DA, Furman JM, Balaban CD. 2005. Motion sickness in migraine sufferers. Expert Opin Pharmacother 6(15): 2691–97.

[110] Marcus et al. 2005.

[111] Marcus et al. 2005.

[112] Marcus et al. 2005.

The dizziness associated with anxiety disorders is not necessarily caused by the anxiety, as is often assumed in clinical practice, but may have a component of disturbed balance control.[113,114] For example, the presence of panic or fear of heights is significantly associated with abnormalities on caloric testing, a form of vestibular testing.[115] A positive result on a questionnaire for Space and Motion Discomfort is significantly associated with abnormality on posturography showing either surface[116] or visual[117] dependence. In testing of vestibulo-ocular reflexes, anxiety patients have been found to have higher vestibular sensitivity or gain than normal controls.[118] Balance assessments of patients diagnosed with panic attacks or agoraphobia (fear of leaving the house) show a high proportion with abnormalities of vestibular function, in some studies greater than 80%, especially if the patients have episodes of dizziness between panic attacks.[119–122]

---

[113] Furman et al. 2005.

[114] Eckhardt-Henn A, Breuer P, Thomalske C, Hoffmann SO, Hopf HC. 2003. Anxiety disorders and other psychiatric subgroups in patients complaining of dizziness. J Anxiety Disord 17(4): 369–88.

[115] Jacob et al. 2009.

[116] Jacob et al. 2009.

[117] Redfern et al. 2007.

[118] Furman JM, Redfern MS, Jacob RG. 2006. Vestibulo-ocular function in anxiety disorders. J Vestib Res 16: 209–15.

[119] Perna G, Dario A, Caldirola D, Stefania B, Cesarani A, Bellodi L. 2001. Panic disorder: the role of the balance system. J Psychiatr Res 35(5): 279–86.

[120] Jacob RG, Furman JM, Durrant JD, Turner SM. 1996. Panic, agoraphobia, and vestibular dysfunction. Am J Psychiatry 153(4): 503–12.

[121] Yardley L, Britton J, Lear S, Bird J, Luxon LM. 1995. Relationship between balance system function and agoraphobic avoidance. Behav Res Ther 33(4): 435–39.

[122] Yardley L, Luxon LM, Lear S, Britton J, Bird J. 1994. Vestibular and posturographic test results in people with symptoms of panic and agoraphobia. J Audiol Med 3: 58–65.

Thus problems with balance function can be due to abnormalities of the inner-ear vestibular organs (utricle, saccule, and semicircular canals) or to abnormal central (brain) integration of balance signals. Mild (mostly central) abnormalities are common and associated with common conditions such as migraine, motion sensitivity, vertigo, and several types of anxiety disorder. People with mild balance abnormalities only feel off balance or insecure in challenging situations where the available sensory information is inadequate or confusing, such as at heights or in the situations described in the questionnaire for Space and Motion Discomfort. The rest of the time, people with mild, compensated balance deficits feel normal and securely oriented in space.

However, if a person is already in a state of adaptation to an ongoing vestibular organ or central balance deficit—even mild, fully compensated deficits—he or she is at particular risk for decompensation with exposure to new balance challenges. Many of the affected people in the present study, I suspect, were in this condition, because their medical histories reveal a variety of risks for mild baseline balance dysfunction. These risks include motion sensitivity, migraine disorder, prior damage to inner-ear organs from industrial noise exposure or chemotherapy, autoimmune disease,[123] fibromyalgia,[124] and normal aging (over 50). We may also consider normal early childhood (age 1–4 or so) as a time of natural mild balance dysfunction[125,126] (see discussion at the end

---

[123] Rinne T, Bronstein AM, Rudge P, Gresty MA, Luxon LM. 1998. Bilateral loss of vestibular function: clinical findings in 53 patients. J Neurol 245(6–7): 314–21.

[124] Rosenhall U, Johansson G, Orndahl G. 1996. Otoneurologic and audiologic findings in fibromyalgia. Scand J Rehabil Med 28(4): 225–32.

[125] Foudriat BA, Di Fabio RP, Anderson JH. 1993. Sensory organization of balance responses in children 3–6 years of age: a normative study with diagnostic implications. Int J Pediatr Otorhinolaryngol 27(3): 255–71.

[126] Steindl R, Kunz K, Schrott-Fischer A, Scholtz AW. 2006. Effect of age and sex on maturation of sensory systems and balance control. Dev Med Child Neurol 48(6): 477–82.

of the next section). Other potential risks for chronic balance deficits, not seen in this study, are whiplash injury and head injury, including concussions and milder head impacts without loss of consciousness,[127–129] and chronic inner-ear conditions such Meniere's disease, dehiscence of the superior semicircular canal, and others.[130]

Cognition and vestibular function

It is now becoming apparent that a variety of cognitive functions depend on coherent vestibular signaling. Clinicians who work with balance-disordered patients are familiar with their struggles with short-term memory, concentration, multitasking, arithmetic, and reading.[131,132] In the perilymphatic fistula syndrome, for example (a form of inner-ear pathology that can follow whiplash, minor head injuries, or pressure trauma to the ear), symptoms of dizziness, headache, stiff neck, and disturbed sleep are accompanied by marked mental performance deficits compared to the patient's baseline.[133] Such cognitive symptoms are difficult to evaluate clinically and are often dismissed as psychological in origin.[134] However, recent research using imaging and other modalities shows that vestibular function exerts a powerful influence over human thinking and memory.

---

[127] Grimm RJ, Hemenway WG, Lebray PR, Black FO. 1989. The perilymph fistula syndrome defined in mild head trauma. Acta Otolaryngol Suppl 464: 1–40.

[128] Ernst A, Basta D, Seidl RO, Todt I, Scherer H, Clarke A. 2005. Management of posttraumatic vertigo. Otolaryngol Head Neck Surg 132(4): 554–58.

[129] Claussen CF, Claussen E. 1995. Neurootological contributions to the diagnostic follow-up after whiplash injuries. Acta Otolaryngol Suppl 520, Pt. 1: 53–56.

[130] Colebatch et al. 1998.

[131] Hanes and McCollum 2006.

[132] Grimm et al. 1989.

[133] Grimm et al. 1989.

[134] Hanes and McCollum 2006.

The vestibular system is ancient in the vertebrate lineage. Hence its neural connections ramify widely in both older and more recently evolved parts of the brain, including the brainstem, midbrain, cerebellum, and occipital, parietal, and frontal cortex.[135] Vestibular injury causes specific cognitive difficulties, but not general cognitive impairment.[136] Vestibular effects on cognition are often attributed to competing stimuli (meaning, challenges to movement and position sense draw attention away from cognitive tasks), but may actually reflect the direct dependence of certain cognitive operations on the vestibular system.[137]

Vestibular input is critical for spatial thinking, body and spatial awareness, spatial memory, and complex spatial or map calculations.[138] Dynamic, active vestibular signaling is needed during the acquisition, storage, and use of information with spatial components, such as building mental maps or deducing a novel path between two points.[139] Patients with 5–10 year histories of bilateral vestibular loss showed marked deficits in a classic experimental task of spatial memory and navigation, accompanied, on average, by a 16.9% volume loss in the hippocampus (a temporal lobe structure essential for learning and memory).[140] In a test of general memory, however, these patients were no different from controls.[141] Vestibular signaling to the hippocampus is known to occur in both humans and other primates via a direct, two-neuron

---

[135] Dieterich M, Brandt T. 2008. Functional brain imaging of peripheral and central vestibular disorders. Brain 131(10): 2538–52.

[136] Hanes and McCollum 2006.

[137] Hanes and McCollum 2006.

[138] Hanes and McCollum 2006.

[139] Brandt T, Schautzer F, Hamilton DA, Bruning R, Markowitsch HJ, Kalla R, Darlington C, Smith P, Strupp M. 2005. Vestibular loss causes hippocampal atrophy and impaired spatial memory in humans. Brain 128: 2732–41.

[140] Brandt et al. 2005.

[141] Brandt et al. 2005.

linkage through the posterior thalamus. There are also other proposed neural pathways.[142]

Disordered vestibular input increases error rates in purely mental tasks based on visualization of remembered objects, showing that coherent vestibular input is critical for thinking successfully and efficiently in spatial terms.[143] This is true even without using sight and beyond the period of memory storage. The tasks included detailed visualization, considered an occipital (visual) cortical task, and mental rotation, a parietal cortical task.[144]

Vestibular stimulation in both humans and other primates activates a variety of areas in the parietal cortex, including 1) a core vestibular processing area (posterior insula), 2) the somatosensory strip, 3) areas involved in hemineglect in stroke patients (ventral parietal), and 4) a region "known to be involved in multimodal coordinate transformations and representation of space" (intraparietal sulcus), which is a principal site for arithmetic and counting tasks.[145]

Hemineglect is a condition after right-sided parietal stroke in which a patient can have so much unawareness of the left side of space that he is oblivious to his own left-sided body parts being paralyzed, for example, or undressed. Vestibular stimulation temporarily corrects or improves this unawareness, in ways that suggest stimulation not only to general attention, but also to cerebral structures involved

---

[142] Brandt et al. 2005.

[143] Mast FW, Merfeld DM, Kosslyn SM. 2006. Visual mental imagery during caloric vestibular stimulation. Neuropsychologia 44(1): 101–9.

[144] Mast et al. 2006. I wonder whether the detailed visualization task also included a parietal component, given the quantitative comparison the subjects had to make with the remembered image.

[145] Hanes and McCollum 2006, p. 82.

in the mental representation of space.[146,147] Vestibular stimulation also improves hemineglect patients' performance on tasks of visual localization and visual-spatial memory retrieval. At baseline, and again 24 hours after the experiment, their responses were biased away from the left side, but this bias was corrected or improved immediately after left vestibular stimulation.[148]

Studies of hemineglect patients have further shown that many mental operations are "spatialized" and dependent on parietal brain areas that have been lost, including mathematical operations involving a "mental number line" with lower numbers on the left,[149,150] clock representations of time,[151] and spelling at the beginnings (left) or ends (right) of words (errors occur opposite to the side of the parietal lesion).[152] In right-handed patients with right parietal strokes, there is no impairment to simple numeric calculation (a left-sided parietal function), but there is impairment to spatialized mathematical thinking, such as finding the midpoint between two numbers.[153] At the other extreme of mental functioning, it has been found that great mathematicians think of numbers in spatial terms,[154] which "may be more efficient because

---

[146] Geminiani G, Bottini G. 1992. Mental representation and temporary recovery from unilateral neglect after vestibular stimulation. J Neurol Neurosurg Psychiatry 55(4): 332–33.

[147] Cappa S, Sterzi R, Vallar G, Bisiach E. 1987. Remission of hemineglect and anosognosia during vestibular stimulation. Neuropsychologia 25: 775–82.

[148] Geminiani and Bottini 1992.

[149] Zorzi M, Priftis K, Umilta C. 2002. Brain damage: neglect disrupts the mental number line. Nature 417: 138–39.

[150] Vuilleumier P, Ortigue S, Brugger P. 2004. The number space and neglect. Cortex 40(2): 399–410.

[151] Vuilleumier et al. 2004.

[152] Hillis HE, Caramazza A. 1995. Spatially specific deficits in processing graphemic representations in reading and writing. Brain Lang 48 (3): 263–308.

[153] Zorzi et al. 2002.

[154] Hadamard J. 1996. *The Mathematician's Mind: The Psychology of Invention in the Mathematical Field*. Princeton University Press, NJ. In Zorzi et al. 2002.

it is grounded in the actual neural representation of numbers."[155] A recent study of outstanding human memorizers shows that spatially oriented strategies are also critical to good memory, by providing an efficient framework for memory organization and retrieval.[156]

Thus current research shows that coherent vestibular neural input is critical for spatialized forms of thinking and memory. Spatialized thinking and memory is intrinsic to many of the things we do with our minds, including mathematical thinking and memory organization (as discussed above) and many forms of map-based or visually based problem-solving or short-term memory we do in everyday life. Spatial thinking is used, for example, to figure out the most efficient path for a set of errands, remember the path and images of the items to be obtained, search for the items on the shelf, and judge if one was given the correct change. It is used for mental "maps" or calendars of one's day, week, or month and its appointments, to picture in three dimensions how to put something together, or imagine what has gone wrong inside a device and initiate a repair. It is used, as well, for understanding the visual clues and images in a movie or TV show. In this context, it is easy to see how vestibular disturbance might impair concentration (which means the ability to perform thinking tasks successfully and efficiently) and memory. Vestibular disturbance also has the potential to affect reading directly, via the reflex control exerted by semicircular canal and otolith organs over eye movements (vestibulo-ocular reflex).

Effects on concentration and memory were nearly ubiquitous in the present study, if one includes all subjects that told me about any problems in this area. For some subjects the deficits were

---

[155] Zorzi et al. 2002.
[156] Maguire EA, Valentine ER, Wilding JM, Kapur N. 2003. Routes to remembering: the brains behind superior memory. Nat Neurosci 6(1): 90–95.

dramatic compared to pre-exposure baseline, including the 7 out of 10 school-age children and teens who showed a decline in their academic performance. Detrimental effects on concentration and memory were significantly associated with normal memory at baseline ($p = 0.027$) and with fatigue and loss of energy and motivation during exposure ($p = 0.018$). Though sleep deprivation/disturbance undoubtedly plays a role in the problems with concentration and memory, qualitative aspects of the mental performance deficiencies suggest a mechanism other than sleep disturbance alone. I propose that this mechanism is the effect of vestibular disturbance on cognition.

It is interesting here to examine a possible role of vestibular disturbance in the learning of very young children, in the toddler and preschool years. Mrs. G (G2) volunteered that her 2½-year-old's (G5) irritability during turbine exposure was especially triggered by her older siblings' "unsteadying her" or coming so close that she thought she might be unsteadied. Children at this age are learning to keep their balance through a variety of different kinds of activities and postures. They are both fascinated and relaxed by vestibular stimulation (swinging, spinning, rolling, somersaults, etc.) and they actively explore the physical world through this play. The behavior of objects in gravity is another source of fascination, starting with babies' casting behavior and moving on to pouring water, sliding down slides, rolling things down inclines, building dams, floating toy boats, blowing bubbles, releasing helium balloons, etc. Vestibular input and processing play a critical role in a) balance during movement, b) the generation, storage, and use of internal maps, and c) recognition of the behavior of objects under the influence of gravity. Indovina et al. measured brain activity by functional MRI in adults as they watched the movement of simulated objects, finding that the vestibular network was selectively engaged when the acceleration of an object was consistent with natural gravity, even though the stimulus was only visual.[157] The authors use this as evidence that "predictive mechanisms of physical laws of motion are represented in the human brain"[158] under the influence of vestibular signaling of the vector of gravity. I suggest that these representations of the physical laws of motion are embedded in the human brain during early childhood as toddlers and children learn through experimentation (play) about the behavior of their bodies and other objects in gravity, and that coherent vestibular signaling is critical to this learning.

Environmental noise, learning, sleep, and health effects

Many studies have quantified the effects of environmental noise on children's learning. Reading acquisition—a language-intensive process—is especially sensitive to the effects of noise in school and at home. The effect is distinct from the effects of noise on attention or working memory,[159] and is correlated with measures of language processing such as speech recognition.[160] Airplane noise, which has a large low frequency component, has a stronger effect than traffic noise in some studies,[161] but traffic noise is also shown to have modest effects on memory in quieter communities.[162] Most studies are cross-sectional, but a longitudinal or cohort study, done

---

[157] Indovina I, Maffei V, Bosco G, Zago M, Macaluso E, Lacquaniti F. 2005. Representation of visual gravitational motion in the human vestibular cortex. Science 308: 416–19.

[158] Indovina et al. 2005.

[159] Haines MM, Stansfeld SA, Job RFS, Berglund B, Head J. 2001. A follow-up study of effects of chronic aircraft noise exposure on child stress responses and cognition. Int J Epidemiol 30: 839–45.

[160] Evans GW, Maxwell L. 1997. Chronic noise exposure and reading deficits: the mediating effects of language acquisition. Environ Behav 29(5): 638–56.

[161] Clark C, Martin R, van Kempen E, Alfred T, Head J, Davies HW, Haines MM, Barrio IL, Matheson M, Stansfeld SA. 2005. Exposure-effect relations between aircraft and road traffic noise exposure at school and reading comprehension: the RANCH project. Am J Epidemiol 163: 27–37.

[162] Lercher P, Evans GW, Meis M. 2003. Ambient noise and cognitive processes among primary schoolchildren. Environ Behav 35(6): 725–35.

when an airport was closed in one location and opened in another, showed similar effects on reading acquisition.[163] One study showed effects of noise on reading and auditory processing in children who lived in an apartment building next to a busy highway. The higher they lived in the building, the quieter were their apartments and the better their reading and auditory discrimination scores (e.g., distinguishing *goat* from *boat*). After controlling for parental education and income, the auditory discrimination scores largely explained the noise-reading linkage.[164] These effects on reading occur at sound levels far less than those needed to produce hearing damage.[165] Children with pre-existing reading deficiencies and children at higher grade levels are more affected, and longer exposure produces larger deficits.[166]

Effects suggestive of wind turbine noise impact on auditory discrimination or central auditory processing were found in the current study. During the period immediately after moving away from turbines and the cessation of her tinnitus, Mrs. A (A2, age 33) found she had a new difficulty understanding conversation in crowded, noisy places. Her son (A3, age 2½) began to confuse several consonant sounds during exposure, and continued to do so in the immediate post-exposure period.

Studies of adults in industrial settings have shown effects of noise on cognitive function when the noise is not considered loud and is nowhere near the threshold for causing damage to hearing. Polish

---

[163] Hygge S, Evans GW, Bullinger M. 2002. A prospective study of some effects of aircraft noise on cognitive performance in schoolchildren. Psychol Sci 13: 469–74.

[164] Cohen S, Glass DC, Singer JE. 1973. Apartment noise, auditory discrimination, and reading ability in children. J Exp Soc Psychol 9: 407–22.

[165] Evans GW. 2006. Child development and the physical environment. Annu Rev Psychol 57: 423–51.

[166] Evans 2006, p. 426.

researchers exposed workers to 50 dBA broadband noise or 50 dBA broadband noise with low frequency components (10-250 Hz) as they worked on standard psychological tests. Low frequency noise impaired performance more than broadband noise without low frequency components, especially in subjects who rated themselves as highly sensitive to low frequency noise. There was no difference in the annoyance ratings for the two types of noise, nor evidence of either habituation or sensitization.[167]

Sleep deprivation is a primary focus of studies of community noise in general and was a major factor for the subjects in the current study. The occurrence of VVVD contributes a distinctive quality to sleep disturbance and to the extent of sleep deprivation near wind turbines, since waking up in a physiologic state of panic leads to prolonged wakefulness or not returning to sleep at all. A second distinctive quality of wind turbine-associated sleep disturbance was nocturia (getting up repeatedly at night to urinate), mostly in adult women, and nocturnal enuresis (bed-wetting) in a 5-year-old girl. Nocturia resolved immediately when subjects slept away from turbines. For the 5-year-old, the enuresis stopped during a family vacation, resumed on return home, and resolved fully when the family moved away.

Studies of whole-body vibration identify 10–18 Hz as frequencies likely to create the urge to urinate,[168] a possible mechanism for nocturia during exposure. Nocturnal enuresis may be a manifestation of the same direct vibratory stimulation in a child not yet developmentally ready to awaken to bladder signals, or it may instead be a parasomnia (like sleep walking, sleep talking, and night terrors) that occurs during disordered partial arousal

---

[167] Pawlaczyk-Luszczynska M, Dudarewicz A, Waszkowska M, Szymczak W, Sliwinska-Kowalska M. 2005. The impact of low-frequency noise on human mental performance. Int J Occup Med Environ Health 18(2): 185–98.

[168] Rasmussen 1982.

from the deeper stages of sleep. Perilymphatic fistula syndrome, a vestibular disorder, includes nocturnal enuresis in adult women in its list of parasomnic manifestations.[169]

Noise at night is known to cause a variety of sleep disturbances, including delay of sleep onset, overt awakening, brief arousals seen on EEG, changes in length and timing of sleep stages, and premature final awakening. Short-term effects of noise during sleep include noise-induced body movements and modifications of autonomic functions such as heart rate, blood pressure, vasoconstriction, and respiratory rate. Noise-induced body movements indicate a low level of arousal from sleep, and occur with noise events as low as 32 dBA. Arousals detected by brain wave pattern on EEG occur with noise events as low as 35 dBA, and conscious awakenings with events of 42 dBA.[170]

Much of the extensive literature on community noise and sleep disturbance focuses on neuroendocrine changes in catecholamine and cortisol levels due to noise disturbance,[171] short-term changes in circulation, including blood pressure, heart rate, cardiac output, and vasoconstriction,[172,173] and the effects of long-

---

[169] Grimm et al. 1989.

[170] Muzet A, Miedema H. 2005. Short-term effects of transportation noise on sleep with specific attention to mechanisms and possible health impact. Draft paper presented at the Third Meeting on Night Noise Guidelines, WHO European Center for Environment and Health, Lisbon, Portugal, April 26–28. Pp. 5–7 in *Report on the Third Meeting on Night Noise Guidelines,* available at www.euro.who.int/Document/NOH/3rd_NNG_final_rep_rev.pdf.

[171] Ising H, Braun C. 2000. Acute and chronic endocrine effects of noise: review of the research conducted at the Institute for Water, Soil and Air Hygiene. Noise Health 7: 7–24.

[172] Babisch W. 2003. Stress hormones in the research on cardiovascular effects of noise. Noise Health 5(18): 1–11.

[173] Babisch W. 2005. Guest editorial: Noise and health. Environ Health Perspect 113(1): A14–15.

term exposure on the risk of myocardial infarction.[174] There is a significant exposure-response relationship between exposure to nighttime aircraft noise, daily average road traffic noise, and hypertension.[175–177]

Most studies of sleep do not differentiate between low frequency and other types of noise, but there is a growing awareness of the particularly disturbing nature of the low frequency components of community noise.[178] One study compared children sleeping with heavy trucks passing two meters from the house walls every two minutes all night long, to children sleeping with traffic noise without the low frequency component. The low frequency noise-exposed children showed increased cortisol production during the first half of the night (an alteration in the normal circadian rhythm of secretion) compared to the other children.[179] Increased cortisol during the first half of the night was significantly related to restless sleep and difficulties in returning to sleep after awakening during the night.

---

[174] Babisch W, Beule B, Schust M, Kersten N, Ising H. 2005. Traffic noise and risk of myocardial infarction. Epidemiology 16(1): 33–40.

[175] Jarup L, Babisch W, Houthuijs D, Pershagen G, Katsouyanni K, Cadum E, Dudley M-L, Savigny P, Seiffert I, Swart W, Breugelmans O, Bluhm G, Selander J, Haralabidis A, Dimakopoulou K, Sourtzi P, Velonakis M, Vigna-Taglianti F. 2008. Hypertension and exposure to noise near airports: the HYENA study. Environ Health Perspect 116(3): 329–33.

[176] Eriksson C, Rosenlund M, Pershagen G, Hilding A, Ostenson C-G, Bluhm G. 2007. Aircraft noise and incidence of hypertension. Epidemiology 18(6): 716–21.

[177] Haralabidis AS, Dimakopoulou K, Vigna-Taglianti F, Giampaolo M, Borgini A, Dudley M-L, Pershagen G, Bluhm G, Houthuijs D, Babisch W, Velonakis M, Katsouyanni K, Jarup L. 2008. Acute effects of night-time noise exposure on blood pressure in populations living near airports. European Heart J 29(5): 658–64.

[178] Persson Waye K. 2004. Effects of low frequency noise on sleep. Noise Health 6(23): 87–91.

[179] Ising H, Ising M. 2002. Chronic cortisol increases in the first half of the night caused by road traffic noise. Noise Health 4: 13–21.

Low frequency noise

Birgitta Berglund, lead editor of the WHO *Guidelines for Community Noise*,[180] stated in a review of low frequency noise effects:

> Although the effects of lower intensities of low-frequency noise are difficult to establish for methodological reasons, evidence suggests that a number of adverse effects of noise in general arise from exposure to low frequency noise: Loudness judgments and annoyance reactions are sometimes reported to be greater for low-frequency noise than other noises for equal sound-pressure level; annoyance is exacerbated by rattle or vibration induced by low-frequency noise; speech intelligibility may be reduced more by low-frequency noise than other noises except those in the frequency range of speech itself, because of the upward spread of masking.
>
> Low-frequency noise (infrasound included) is the superpower of the frequency range: It is attenuated less by walls and other structures; it can rattle walls and objects; it masks higher frequencies more than it is masked by them; it crosses great distances with little energy loss due to atmospheric and ground attenuation; ear protection devices are much less effective against it; it is able to produce resonance in the human body; and it causes greater subjective reactions (in the laboratory and in the community studies) and to some extent physiological reactions in humans than mid- and high frequencies.[181]

---

[180] World Health Organization. 1999. *Guidelines for Community Noise*, ed. Berglund B, Lindvall T, Schwela DH. 159 pp. www.who.int/docstore/peh/noise/guidelines2.html

[181] Berglund B, Hassmen P, Job RFS. 1996. Sources and effects of low frequency noise. J Acoust Soc Am 99(5): 2985–3002, p. 2985.

> Low-frequency noise also differs from other noise in producing vibrations of the human body and other objects.... Motion sickness has been linked to low-frequency noise even without accompanying vibration.[182]

Many subjects in the present study stated that turbine noise was different from other types of noise, using words like "invasive" and "unnatural," and saying that it was impossible to get used to this noise. Several said it wouldn't sound loud to people who did not live at their homes, or they described a "swish" or "hum" as extremely bothersome noises. A number spoke favorably of living near heavily traveled roads or urban train lines, compared to living near wind turbines. All who moved, moved into villages, towns, or suburbs, where there was more traffic but no danger of turbines being built next to them. The descriptions make it clear that there is a disturbing quality about turbine noise which is more than its audible loudness and that, over time, people become sensitized to wind turbine noise, rather than get used to it.

In the present study, Mr. and Mrs. G described a resonance or standing wave phenomenon in one room of their turbine-exposed home. At one end of this room, Mrs. G felt internal vibration, even though she could not feel any surfaces or objects vibrating when she put her hand on them. Mr. G felt peculiar in the same place, and always had to walk quickly away from that spot before his feeling progressed to nausea. In the home of family C, an audiologist detected vibration in the floor of a small room the family identified as having the worst problem in the home, and felt nauseated when he put his forehead against it.[183]

---

[182] Berglund et al. 1996, p. 2993.

[183] Personal communication from acoustician; name withheld for confidentiality reasons.

At a NASA test facility in the 1960's, healthy young men were exposed to low frequency noise in the 1–50 Hz frequency range at 110 to 150 dB for 2–3 minutes (high amplitude and short duration). Over the full 1–50 Hz frequency range they experienced fatigue and took longer to perform assigned tasks. At frequencies less than 25 Hz there was an "annoying tickling" in the ear. In the same frequency range, there were modulations of speech, moderate vibrations of the chest, and fullness in the hypopharynx with an annoying gag sensation. "In regard to the opinions of those tested, it was indicated that the sensations involved were impressive."[184]

A case that was similar to the cases presented in this paper involved a couple in Germany in 1996. After moving into a new house outside a provincial city, the couple experienced symptoms with increasing intensity, including "indisposition, decrease in performance, sleep disturbance, headache, ear pressure, crawl parasthesy,[185] or shortness of breath."[186] Their case was intensely investigated with both A-weighted and linear measurements of noise indoors and outdoors, correlated in real time with the couple's symptoms. In time, the symptoms were correlated with intensity of noise below 10 Hz. The couple's symptoms and the intensity of noise below 10 Hz both varied with the wind and weather, and were worse in the winter. No plausible mechanism for production of such noises or correspondences to local sources of noise, such as the housing complex heating plant, was found. Symptoms occurred when the sound pressure level at 1 Hz was 65 dB, well

---

[184] Edge PM, Mayes WH. 1966. Description of Langley low-frequency noise facility and study of human response to noise frequencies below 50 cps. NASA Technical Note, NASA TN D-3204. 11 pp.

[185] *Paresthesia* means a prickling sensation, the "pins and needles," felt when a numb foot is waking up. I interpret "crawl parasthesy" to mean a sensation like insects crawling on the skin or in the chest. One of the current study's subjects, I2, also described "pins and needles" inside her chest.

[186] Feldmann J, Pitten FA. 2004. Effects of low-frequency noise on man: a case study. Noise Health 7(25): 23–28.

below hearing threshold. None of the frequencies responsible for the symptoms, all below 10 Hz, had sound pressure levels above 80 dB. The decibel levels that affected the man and wife in their home were far less than their own threshold hearing levels measured in a sound lab. The authors hypothesized that infrasound, with its very long wavelengths (10 Hz, for example, has a 34 m wavelength in air), causes strong pressure fluctuations in relatively small closed rooms—pressure fluctuations that are detected more by the whole body and its inner organs than by the ears.

Similar intensive investigations, using linear as well as A-weighted sound levels, 1/3 octave sound pressure levels down to 1 Hz, indoor measurements, and assessments of wall vibration, have proved fruitful in other low frequency noise complaint investigations.[187] These investigators, from a state environmental agency in Germany, paid attention to spontaneous statements by the affected people, to see whether perceptions of noise followed a systematic pattern. They found that "noises which in many cases induced vehement complaints were to a large extent of rather low sound levels,"[188] and that indoor ventilator noise and noises generated by structure-borne sound transmission were distinctly more disturbing than road traffic noise. These authors documented standing waves in rooms by measuring and comparing loudness in dBA and dB(lin) at the center of the room and near walls. They detected vibration in walls, and correlated the dominant frequency and its corresponding wavelength to the size of the room in discussing how a standing wave was established in the room.

For this kind of complaint, the authors noted,

---

[187] Findeis H, Peters E. 2004. Disturbing effects of low-frequency sound immissions and vibrations in residential buildings. Noise Health 6(23): 29–35.

[188] Findeis and Peters 2004, p. 29.

More than half... were made on the grounds of sleep disturbance. Quite often symptoms like "a roaring in the head, especially when lying down" were brought forward. Time and again, "a feeling of riding a lift [elevator]" was reported, and over and again the measuring team had the impression that the reported immissions [noise] meant a nerve-wracking experience for the exposed persons. Several complainants even got into a state of being aggressive. There were reports by a number of trustworthy persons on how they at first—for instance when moving into the flat—did not even notice any immissions. But in the course of a few weeks they began to perceive them distinctly and [the immissions] became intolerable after continued exposure. It was obvious that in these cases the sensibility of specific noise components had developed. Thus, it is understandable that non-exposed persons were at a difficulty to even acknowledge such noise immissions.[189]

Wind turbines produce noise in the low and infrasonic frequency ranges. The issue has not been whether they produce low frequency or infrasonic noise, but whether the amplitudes are sufficient to cause human effects. According to data published by van den Berg,[190] unweighted amplitudes at 1 Hz, at one wind park under one set of weather conditions, were in the 70–100 dB range, declining to the 55–75 dB range at 10 Hz and the 50–60 dB range at 100 Hz. Wind turbine noise has a pulsating quality, produced as the airfoil blades swing past the tower, compressing the air between blade and tower. These low frequency pressure fluctuations, among other effects, modify the loudness of the higher frequency sounds coming from the turbines, producing the audible "swish"

---

[189] Findeis and Peters 2004, p. 32.

[190] van den Berg 2004a.

that synchronizes with the feeling of pulsation some subjects felt in their chests. Coming from several towers at once, these low frequency air pressure fluctuations may synchronize and reinforce, depending on the orientation of the towers and house and the timing of the individual turbines. Three families in this study (A, B, and F) lived in houses nearly in line with a row of turbines. For families A and B, the area's worst storms, "nor'easters," swept right down the line towards their houses, which were built on a hill at the level of the turbine hubs. These two families, though they were a kilometer (about 3300 feet) from the closest of the 10 turbines, moved out faster—in five months—than any of the other families, and had particularly severe symptoms.

Studies of turbine noise also show that noise carries farther than predicted by conventional industry modeling. This has to do not only with the low frequency components of the noise, which attenuate less with distance, but also with layering of the atmosphere at night, which creates cool still air at ground level and brisk, laminar airflow at turbine hub heights.[191] Industry models do not take these factors into account. Nor do they allow for a noise source more than 30 m above the ground. (Turbine hub heights in this study were 59–90 m.) Nor do they allow for increased transmission of sound in front of and behind the blades (with less sound transmission in the plane of the blades, including under the turbines), sky reflections, or weather conditions that focus the noise transmissions.[192]

Vibroacoustic Disease (VAD) model
High intensities of low frequency noise over prolonged time periods may cause marked neurologic damage, as described

---

[191] van den Berg 2004b.

[192] Richard James, INCE Full Member, personal communication, 5/11/08.

by the Vibroacoustic Disease (VAD) group in Portugal.[193] This is a provocative body of research, full of interesting case descriptions and pathology studies, but compromised by absence of specified study group criteria, absence of control groups, and lack of quantification. The study group consists of 140 aircraft maintenance and repair technicians in the Portuguese Air Force, of whom 22 (15.7%) had adult-onset epilepsy, compared to a national prevalence of 0.2%.[194] Some of the case descriptions of the subjects with epilepsy also include cognitive decline, depression, paranoia, and rage attacks.[195] The descriptions are similar to those of retired professional football players with histories of multiple concussions.[196,197] The vibroacoustic disease researchers ascribe VAD pathology to whole-body vibration induced by the noise, with the pathology of each body part induced by vibration of that part. Neurologic effects may be due to neuronal or axonal shearing, as in the multiple concussions scenario, or due to microangiopathy in the brain, meaning, effects on and occlusion of small blood vessels.[198]

With regard to the chest, the VAD researchers have used human autopsy and biopsy and animal rearing studies to describe loss of

---

[193] Castelo Branco and Alves-Pereira 2004.

[194] Castelo Branco and Alves-Pereira 2004.

[195] Martinho Pimenta AJ, Castelo Branco NAA. 1999. Neurological aspects of vibroacoustic disease. Aviat Space Environ Med 70(3): A91–95.

[196] Omalu BI, DeKosky ST, Minster RL, Kamboh MI, Hamilton RL, Wecht CH. 2005. Chronic traumatic encephalopathy in a National Football League player. Neurosurgery 57: 128–34.

[197] Omalu BI, DeKosky ST, Hamilton RL, Minster RL, Kamboh MI, Shakir AM, Wecht CH. 2006. Chronic traumatic encephalopathy in a National Football League player: part II. Neurosurgery 59: 1086–93.

[198] Martinho Pimenta and Castelo Branco 1999.

cilia and microvilli from epithelial surfaces of the bronchi,[199-201] pleura,[202] and pericardium.[203] They also describe thickening of bronchial epithelial basement membrane,[204] pericardium,[205] and blood vessel walls[206] by extra, organized collagen and elastin. Several of the animal-rearing studies on bronchial epithelial changes are well controlled and convincing.[207,208]

Based on the vibroacoustic disease research, I hypothesize that vibratory or pulsating air pressure fluctuations in subjects' airways in the present study may induce shearing of surface cilia, thus impairing the clearance of mucus and particulates from airways. This in turn could make subjects more susceptible to lower respiratory infections and increased airway irritation and reactivity (asthma). The Eustachian tube and middle ear could be susceptible

---

[199] Oliveira MJR, Pereira AS, Ferreira PG, Guinaraes L, Freitas D, Carvalho APO, Grande NR, Aguas AP. 2004. Arrest in ciliated cell expansion on the bronchial lining of adult rats caused by chronic exposure to industrial noise. Environ Res 97: 282–86.

[200] Oliveira MJR, Pereira AS, Castelo Branco NAA, Grande NR, Aguas AP. 2002. In utero and postnatal exposure of Wistar rats to low frequency/high intensity noise depletes the tracheal epithelium of ciliated cells. Lung 179: 225–32.

[201] Monteiro M, Ferreira JR, Alves-Pereira M, Castelo Branco NAA. 2007. Bronchoscopy in vibroacoustic disease I: "pink lesions." Inter-Noise 2007, August 28–31, Istanbul, Turkey.

[202] Pereira AS, Grande NR, Monteiro E, Castelo Branco MSN, Castelo Branco NAA. 1999. Morphofunctional study of rat pleural mesothelial cells exposed to low frequency noise. Aviat Space Environ Med 70(3): A78–85.

[203] Castelo Branco NAA, Aguas AP, Pereira AS, Monteiro E, Fragata JIG, Tavares F, Grande NR. 1999. The human pericardium in vibroacoustic disease. Aviat Space Environ Med 70(3): A54–62.

[204] Castelo Branco NAA, Monteiro M, Ferreira JR, Monteiro E, Alves-Pereira M. 2007. Bronchoscopy in vibroacoustic disease III: electron microscopy. Inter-Noise 2007, August 28–31, Istanbul, Turkey.

[205] Castelo Branco et al. 1999.

[206] Castelo Branco NAA. 1999. A unique case of vibroacoustic disease: a tribute to an extraordinary patient. Aviat Space Environ Med 70(3): A27–31.

[207] Oliveira et al. 2004.

[208] Oliveira et al. 2002.

to the same process, leading to prolonged middle ear effusions and unusual acute infections.

The increased asthma seen in subjects F1 and F3 may also have a connection to their frequent use of paracetemol (acetaminophen) for headaches during turbine exposure.[209]

Community noise studies and *annoyance*
Studies of community noise frequently assess a quality called *annoyance*. "Apart from 'annoyance,'" the World Health Organization writes, "people may feel a variety of negative emotions when exposed to community noise, and may report anger, disappointment, dissatisfaction, withdrawal, helplessness, depression, anxiety, distraction, agitation, or exhaustion."[210]

Beyond even these negative emotions, moving out of an owned home indicates that people feel sick and under threat, judging that their survival and well-being, and that of their children, will be enhanced by moving out—even as they exhaust limited resources to do so and face unrecompensed loss of their major asset, their home.

Sick and *annoyed* are not the same thing. In English, *annoyance* carries an air of triviality, like a mosquito buzzing around one's head. *Sickness* threatens survival itself.

Pedersen and Persson Waye assessed annoyance (which may be a shorthand for the above list of negative emotions, but remains different from sickness) among 351 households near wind turbines in Sweden in 2000. They used a mailed survey and compared annoyance to modeled A-weighted sound pressure levels they

---
[209] Beasley et al. 2008.
[210] World Health Organization 1999, *Guidelines for Community Noise*, p. 50.

calculated to exist outside homes near clusters of one to five turbines of power 0.15–0.65 MW (much smaller than in the current study), based on the homes' distances from turbines.[211] They found people to be highly annoyed by wind turbine noise at sound pressure levels much lower than for other types of community noise. The A-weighted decibel level (in a measure averaged and weighted over time, L_{eq}) that corresponded to 15% of the people being highly annoyed was 38 dBA for wind turbines, 57 dBA for aircraft, 63 dBA for road traffic, and 70 dBA for railways. The curve for annoyance due to wind turbine noise had a steep slope, so that by 41 dBA, 35% of people were *highly annoyed*. Sixteen percent of respondents over 35 dBA reported that their sleep was disturbed by wind turbine noise.

I interpret this result as an indication of the degree to which wind turbine noise has a disturbing quality not captured by its A-weighted measurement. Since A-weighting emphasizes higher frequencies and filters out lower frequencies, the qualitative difference may be related to the presence of low frequency components. Even without directly measuring the low frequency components, this study is potentially useful with regard to regulating noise and determining setback distances for turbines. Since the study was done in units of dBA outside houses, and most community noise regulations (including for wind turbines) also use units of dBA outside houses, we can easily translate this result into the recommendation that wind turbine ordinances need to limit the turbine noise levels outside houses to less than 35 dBA. This does not mean that only 35 dB of real noise is present, but rather that in the common measurement unit of community noise—which is dBA—35 is a number that represents a significant amount

---

[211] Pedersen E, Persson Waye K. 2004. Perception and annoyance due to wind turbine noise: a dose-response relationship. J Acoust Soc Am 116(6): 3460–70.

of sleep disturbance and high annoyance if the noise comes from wind turbines.

In a continuation study that involved interviewing participants, Pedersen found that some people had moved out of their homes, rebuilt their homes in an attempt to exclude turbine noise, or begun legal proceedings because of problems associated with turbine exposure.[212] Pedersen and Persson Waye also found informants who were sensitive to both noise and blade motion, felt violated or invaded by turbine noise, and found their houses to be places where they could no longer find restoration[213]—qualitative similarities to the current study.

Van den Berg, Pedersen, and colleagues conducted another survey study of noise and annoyance in the Netherlands in 2007.[214] They mailed questionnaires to 1960 households within 2.1 km (1.3 mi) of at least two adjacent 0.5–3 MW turbines, with 725 responses (37% response rate). The questionnaire asked about visual and auditory perceptions, economic benefit, annoyance, chronic diseases, current symptoms, psychological stress, and sleep disturbance, and looked at variation in these factors (as in the Swedish study) against modeled A-weighted noise levels.

Though it contained several questions about health, this study was not properly constructed to sample health in an accurate or realistic way. The evidence for this is found in the study results themselves, which contain significant bias or skew relative to known health parameters.

---

[212] Pedersen 2007.

[213] Pedersen and Persson Waye 2007.

[214] van den Berg et al. 2008b.

For example, 2% of respondents in this study indicated that they had chronic migraine disorder.[215] The population prevalence of migraine disorder is remarkably stable across countries and time when controlled for age, sex, and definition of the disease, being 5–6% for males and 15–18% for females.[216,217] A finding of 2% is an underestimate, indicating that something about this study's method of sampling migraine prevalence was awry.

Sampling and sampling error occur at several levels, such as the level of selecting respondents and the level of sampling the respondents' thoughts through questioning. Potential flaws at each level can be identified in this study.

First, the researchers attempted to elicit objective health information with just two questions in this survey, one on past or underlying health and one on current symptoms. (Separate questions addressed sleep disturbance.) This is the single question about underlying health:

> 37. Do you have any long term/chronic disease? (no → 38, yes). *If yes, which chronic disease do you have?* (diabetes, high blood pressure, tinnitus, hearing impairment, cardiovascular disease, migraine, other *viz*:)[218]

This is a very brief and superficial question, and it is not surprising that it failed to capture all the diagnoses of migraine that should have been present in a random population sample. In medical

---

[215] van den Berg et al. 2008b, p. 48.

[216] Lipton RB, Bigal ME, Diamond M, Freitag F, Reed ML, Stewart WF; AMPP Advisory Group. 2007. Migraine prevalence, disease burden, and the need for preventive therapy. Neurology 68(5): 343–49.

[217] Stewart WF, Simon D, Shechter A, Lipton RB. 1995. Population variation in migraine prevalence: a meta-analysis. J Clin Epidemiol 48(2): 269–80.

[218] van den Berg et al. 2008b, Appendix p. 5.

research, in contrast, the presence or absence of a diagnosis in a subject is established by multiple proven and validated questions directly tied to the formal definition of the illness, administered by a trained interviewer. Even in clinical practice, which is less formal, an accurate review of systems still requires a series of specific screening questions and the knowledge of when and how to question in further depth. No clinician or health researcher would rely on a question like the above to elicit full and accurate information about the past health history.

The same question also failed to elicit accurate prevalence figures for tinnitus. Tinnitus prevalence among survey respondents was 2%, whereas 4% is the likely population-level figure for the respondents' average age of 54.[219] Tinnitus prevalence also did not show age differences in this sample,[220] whereas in reality tinnitus has a well-documented pattern of increasing prevalence with advancing age.[221]

The question's time frame is also unclear. Were the authors trying to find out about baseline susceptibilities (health conditions before turbines) or did they hypothesize that exposure to wind turbines might alter the prevalence of these chronic conditions? Though they never state it explicitly, their analysis makes it clear they hypothesized that health effects due to wind turbines, if they exist, would present as higher levels of the listed chronic diseases closer to wind turbines.[222] To think that they might find such an effect with this type of sample size and mode of study verges on silly, it is

---

[219] National Institute on Deafness and Other Communication Disorders, USA, website, "Prevalence of chronic tinnitus." 2009. www.nidcd.nih.gov/health/statistics/prevalence.htm

[220] van den Berg et al. 2008b, p. 47.

[221] National Institute on Deafness and Other Communication Disorders, "Prevalence of chronic tinnitus." 2009.

[222] van den Berg et al. 2008b, p. 50.

so far outside the parameters of how such issues are studied (see, for example, studies cited in footnotes 171–177, above). As a result, this study's failure to find such an effect is meaningless.

There were also sampling problems at the level of subject selection. First, the study has no control population that is not exposed to turbine noise. It samples within 2.1 km (1.3 mi) of turbines, using the unspoken assumption that the people at the outer edge of this radius will not be exposed to significant amounts of turbine noise and can therefore act as a control group. An epidemiologic study, in contrast, would have a control group of households subjected to all the same procedures for household selection, questioning, and noise modeling as the study group, but without turbines present.

Second, uncontrolled subject selection processes occurred at the level of the household. Once questionnaires reached households, what happened? Nearly two-thirds of households declined to respond. The researchers studied a subset of non-responders using a very brief questionnaire that yielded a modestly higher (48%) response rate. The brief questionnaire showed that non-responders were similar to responders in their average degree of annoyance at wind turbine noise, but did not address the issue of whether non-responders differed from responders in health parameters.

An additional process of self-selection occurred within responder households, since only one individual replied and only answered questions about himself. The householders chose who replied. On a very mundane and human level, we can imagine how this process might have selected against migraineurs in the sample, if the person with a headache the day the survey arrived asked someone else to fill it out.

The survey's second question about health concerned current symptoms, as follows:

38. Have you been troubled by the following symptoms during the last months? ((almost) never, at least once a month, at least once a week, (almost) daily) [sic]

> Headache
> Undue tiredness
> Pain and stiffness in the back, neck or shoulders
> Feeling tense or stressed
> Depressivity
> Not very sociable, wanting to be alone
> Irritable
> Resigned
> Fearful
> Concentration problems
> Nausea
> Vertigo
> Mood changes
> Other, namely: *(please indicate what)*[223]

This is an odd list of "symptoms"—an undifferentiated mix of physical and psychological, with a few simple "feeling words" thrown in. It does not make sense as a symptom list—not without more detail and structuring into symptom groups. As with the chronic disease question, above, medical researchers and clinicians know that accurate and complete information cannot be elicited in this format, especially about delicate subjects like mood states and health. This question, too, is unclear about timing—pre-existing vs. during exposure, while near turbines or away from them.

This question in fact yielded little information that was useful to the researchers. In their analysis, the only reference to the health symptoms question is as follows:

---

[223] van den Berg et al. 2008b, Appendix p. 6.

> Respondents who did not benefit economically from wind turbines reported more chronic diseases and health symptoms than those who benefited.... The observed differences between the sub-samples regarding chronic diseases and health symptoms could be due to age effects; respondents who did not benefit economically were older than those who benefited.[224]

Otherwise, through a long and detailed statistical analysis of stress, sleep disturbance, noise, annoyance, and chronic disease, the health symptoms question does not appear again.

The researchers expanded their questioning on mood states by incorporating a screening interview for mental illness used in general medical practice, called the General Health Questionnaire.[225] Despite the name, it is not a health questionnaire, nor is it a measure of psychological stress (which is how the authors use it). The GHQ-12 is a screening tool for mental illness, used to help a physician figure out which of his presenting patients need assessment for psychiatric illness. It was validated (meaning compared against other effective means of diagnosis to see if it identified the right people) for its declared purpose, not as a measure of psychological stress. The authors present it as a "validated instrument" for "measuring 'perceived health,'"[226] then use it in their analysis as a measure of "psychological stress," morphing the question set from one purpose to another to another without justification.[227]

---

[224] van den Berg et al. 2008b, p. 49.

[225] Goldberg DP, Hillier VF. 1979. A scaled version of the General Health Questionnaire. Psychol Med 9(1): 139–45. The 28-item GHQ may be found at http://www.gp-training.net/protocol/docs/ghq.doc and the 12-item GHQ (used by van den Berg et al.) at www.webpoll.org/psych/GHQ12.htm.

[226] van den Berg et al. 2008b, p. 20.

[227] van den Berg et al. 2008b, p. 47.

In the Dutch survey study results, owners of turbines lived the closest to turbines and were able to turn them off if they or their neighbors were bothered by the noise—a key difference between the Netherlands and other countries. These closer respondents tended to be farmers and to benefit economically from the turbines. They were on average younger, healthier, and, as it happens, better educated than the respondents living farther from turbines.

Sleep disturbance, annoyance, and questionnaire measures of stress were correlated with noise levels among people who did not benefit economically from turbines. Annoyance occurred at lower dBA noise levels than for road, rail, or air traffic noise, as in the similar Swedish study. Being awakened from sleep was associated with higher noise levels, and difficulty falling asleep and higher stress scores were associated with annoyance. "Respondents with economic benefits reported almost no annoyance,"[228] though they lived closest to the turbines and experienced the highest modeled noise levels. If turbine owners were turning the turbines off when they were bothered or during sleep, then the modeled noise levels would not have accurately represented real noise levels close to the turbines.

Despite health being inadequately sampled in this study, the authors still draw conclusions that are interpreted popularly as evidence against health effects by wind turbines, in sentences like this one from the authors' summary: "There is no indication that the sound from wind turbines had an effect on respondents' health, except for the interruption of sleep."[229] Though it is downplayed in this sentence, sleep interruption is in fact of great significance to health. The authors are remiss in failing to acknowledge that the study methods do not have the power to detect other health effects.

---

[228] van den Berg et al. 2008b, Summary, p. ii.
[229] van den Berg et al. 2008b, Summary, p. ii.

The authors would have more accurately captured the survey's health results had they written, "Sleep disturbance or interruption, an effect of profound importance to health, was correlated with turbine noise levels. Unfortunately, the survey could not effectively address other health questions due to bias introduced at the level of data collection. An important finding is the possibility of biased responses from respondents benefiting economically from turbines, yet it is equally possible that turbine owners are in the habit of turning turbines off at critical times, thus avoiding both annoyance and sleep disturbance."

Recommendations

For physicians practicing near wind turbine installations, I suggest incorporating proximity to turbines into the personal and social history in a neutral and non-suggestive way, especially for the types of symptoms described in this report.

With regard to turbine setback from dwellings: in Table 1B we see that the subjects in the current study lived between 305 m (1000 ft) and 1.5 km (4900 ft or 0.93 mi) from the closest turbine. There were three severely affected families at 930–1000 m (3000–3300 ft) from turbines. This study suggests that communities that allow 305–457 m (1000–1500 ft) setbacks from homes, like those in New York State, may have families who need to move after turbines go into operation.

All turbine ordinances, I believe, should establish mechanisms to ensure that turbine developers will buy out any affected family at the full pre-turbine value of their home, so that people are not trapped between unlivable lives and destitution through home abandonment. By shifting the burden of this expense to turbine developers, I would hope that developers might have a stronger incentive to improve their techniques for noise prediction and to accept noise level criteria recommended by such agencies as the World Health Organization and the International Standards Organization,[230] and fortified by the findings of Pedersen (above).

With regard to families already affected, developers and permitting agencies share the responsibility for turbines built too close to homes, and together need to provide the financial means for these families to re-establish their lives at their previous level of health, comfort, and prosperity.

I support the recommendations for noise level criteria and procedures for noise monitoring by George Kamperman and Richard James.[231] A single setback distance may not be both protective and fair in all environments with all types of turbines, but it is clear, from the current study and others, that minimum protective distances need to be more than the 1–1.5 km (3280–4900 ft or 0.62–0.93 mi) at which there were severely affected subjects in this study, more than the 1.6 km (5250 ft or 1 mi) at which there were affected subjects in Dr. Harry's UK study,[232] and, in mountainous terrain, more than the 2–3.5 km (1.24–2.2 mi) at which there were symptomatic subjects in Professor Robyn Phipps's New Zealand study.[233]

Two kilometers, or 1.24 miles, remains the baseline shortest setback from residences (and hospitals, schools, nursing homes, etc.) that communities should consider. In mountainous terrain, 2 miles (3.2 km) is probably a better guideline.

---

[230] See Kamperman and James 2008b.

[231] Kamperman and James 2008b. Presented in shorter form, Kamperman GW, James RR. 2008a. Simple guidelines for siting wind turbines to prevent health risks. Noise-Con, July 28–31, annual conference of the Institute of Noise Control Engineering/USA.

[232] Harry 2007.

[233] Phipps 2007.

Setbacks may well need to be longer than these minima, as guided by the noise criteria developed by Kamperman and James.

Suggestions for further research

- Epidemiologic studies comparing populations exposed and not exposed to wind turbines with regard to the prevalence of specific symptoms, such as tinnitus and balance complaints. Such studies might be best conducted in European countries that have both national health data systems and significant numbers of wind turbines.
- Case series by neurotologists internationally, who are able to do appropriate objective examinations and testing in addition to clinical history.
- Collaboration between physicians and independent noise engineers to find which specific frequencies and intensities of sound and vibration correlate with subjects' symptoms in real time, and to establish a standard protocol for wind turbine noise sampling that includes these specific frequencies and intensities of sound and vibration.
- Further clinical/laboratory research on the effects of low frequency noise and vibration on the human vestibular system.
- Case control studies by specialist physicians near turbine installations on rarer associated symptoms, such as ocular problems, lower respiratory infections, asthma, persistent middle ear effusions, failure of anticoagulation, loss of diabetes control, exacerbation of arrhythmias, and exacerbation of gastrointestinal conditions.
- Studies of turbine noise and children's learning. Standardized test scores, before and after turbines are built near schools or in a community, might be compared to test scores of similar,

non-exposed schools and communities across the same years. The current study suggests that both school and home turbine noise exposures would have to be quantified.

Limitations of the study

- The study was done by interview and only limited medical records were available. Physical exam and appropriate testing (such as hearing, balance, and neuropsychological testing) would clarify and provide objective evidence for otologic and neurologic problems. Physical exam and appropriate testing are necessary to assess the rarer associated conditions not included in the core symptoms of Wind Turbine Syndrome.

- Participant memory limitations or distortions. I excluded several families from the analysis because they were unclear about what had happened when, combined with not having spent enough time in a post-exposure situation. I insisted on a post-exposure period to compensate for the difficulty of accurately comparing before-exposure experience to the current situation of exposure.

- Minimization or exaggeration of effects. I felt some subjects may have minimized potentially embarrassing or frightening issues, such as nocturia in men and cognitive difficulties in general. In other families, excluded from the analysis, one spouse was clearly committed to staying in the house and minimized what the other spouse said. I endeavored to protect against exaggeration by including in the study only families who had moved out of their homes or done something else expensive in response to their symptoms, proving their symptom severity in ways other than words. The one exception to this rule was the family of an American physician and nurse, whose professionalism, I felt, was protective.

- The study was limited to English-speaking subjects. There was only one non-native speaker. He was competent at English and had an English-speaking wife, but there may have been subtleties in his symptoms that he didn't tell me about.
- Small case series sample. For this study, I chose a cluster of the most severely affected and most articulate subjects I could find. It is not a large enough sample to establish a gradient of effects with a gradient of exposure (distance from the turbines). It is not an epidemiologic sample that could establish prevalence of effects within exposure gradients or according to age or pre-existing conditions. Conditions that occurred in one or a few study subjects require case-control studies and cannot be established as part of the syndrome from this study.
- Limited duration of follow-up. For cognitive symptoms improved but not resolved at the post-exposure interview, the time course of resolution is not clear.

THREE

The CASE HISTORIES: The raw data

Case History A1 (page 1 of 2)

Person Mr. A

Age 32

Pre-exposure health status Good

Health history No significant

Previous noise exposure Diesel fishing boat from childhood

Time to onset of symptoms Immediate with progression

	Pre-exposure	During exposure*	Post-exposure**
Sleep	Good but always easily awakened by noise.	"I didn't really." Hard to fall asleep. Frequent awakening due to child's frequent awakening.	Good, at baseline. Child sleeping through night.
Headache	Rare, mild	Continuous headache at home which resolved after several hours away and resumed several hours after return, with onset 3 weeks into turbine start-up process. OTC and prescription analgesics, addition of glasses not helpful.	Resolved
Cognition	Normal. Runs own fishing business. Mild difficulty with memory, especially for names and faces.	Memory problems: "You'd think I was 99." When arriving at a store or storage building, could not remember what he had come to get without a list.	Partial recovery: self-rated memory 80–85% at baseline, 2% during exposure, and 10% at 6 weeks after moving
Mood	Good. Usually does not show annoyance.	Loss of usual energy and enjoyment for spring fishing season. Mildly irritable.	Anger about home abandonment, otherwise resolved.
Balance/equilibrium	Normal, never carsick or seasick	"A little shaky on feet every now and then" at home.	Resolved
Ear/hearing	Mild subjective hearing loss attributed to diesel engine exposure, no tinnitus	Repetitive popping in ears for first 3 weeks. Tinnitus started several weeks after headache onset and worsened over time.	Resolved

Case History A1 (page 2 of 2)

	Pre-exposure	During exposure*	Post-exposure**
Eye/vision	Normal without glasses	Burning sensation in eyes. When headache and tinnitus were severe, eyes "felt like they were going to fall out on the table if you looked down." Had normal eye exam.	Resolved
Other neurological	Normal, mild concussion age 14	No change	No change
Cardiovascular	Normal including BP (110–120/80 in 2006)	Mild diastolic hypertension on one reading (128/94 on 4/4/07)	No further BP measurements obtained.
Gastrointestinal	Normal	Nausea when headache was severe. No vomiting or other gastrointestinal changes.	Resolved
Respiratory	Normal except smokes	No change	No change
Other		"You feel different up there, draggy, worn out before you even start anything." "It was a chore to walk across the yard." Symptoms were present in all wind directions, better during rain, and worse with wind from direction of turbines or from the 180-degree opposite direction.	When visiting family 100 km away, "I felt better all over, like you could do a cartwheel." Feels well at new house.

*Exposure period 5 months.
**Interviewed 6 weeks after move.

Case History A2 (page 1 of 2)

Person
Mrs. A

Age
33

Pre-exposure health status
Good. Pregnant during exposure and delivered at term 4 days before moving.

Health history
Polycystic ovarian syndrome and metabolic syndrome. Caesarian section for first delivery.

Previous noise exposure
Worked at biomedical chemical plant for 5 years with 1–2 hours/week exposure to noisy areas.

Time to onset of symptoms
Immediate with progression

	Pre-exposure	During exposure*	Post-exposure**
Sleep	Normal. Sleeps through noises other than children.	Frequent awakening	Normal, resolved
Headache	Rare, mild	Occasional headache	At baseline
Cognition	Concentration "great," works as accountant	Noticed concentration problem at work when training someone; working to focus; trainee had to help	Resolved
Mood	Good, including during and after first pregnancy	Irritable	Resolved
Balance/equilibrium	Gets seasick but not carsick	Slight unsteadiness	Resolved
Ear/hearing	Normal hearing. Persistent middle ear fluid in late 20's, resolved. Tinnitus in past when emerging from noisy plant.	Repetitive popping in ears and decreased hearing for first 3 weeks, then tinnitus began. Tinnitus varied with exposure and worsened over time.	Tinnitus resolved, but has new difficulty understanding conversation in a noisy room. Has to watch speaker's face.
Eye/vision	Wears glasses. Eyes water if strained.	No change	No change
Other neurological	Normal, no concussion	No change	No change
Cardiovascular	Normal except h/o temporary stress-related hypertension at age 22.	Normal	Normal
Gastrointestinal	Nausea and GER during pregnancy	No change	Resolved after delivery

Case History A2 (page 2 of 2)

	Pre-exposure	During exposure*	Post-exposure**
Respiratory	Normal, no asthma or smoking.	Lower respiratory infection for 6 weeks not treated until after delivery and move.	Resolved
Other		"Not noisy like a chainsaw, more like pulsating annoyance. To another person it wouldn't sound loud."	
Animals		Dog barks at windmills and up more at night.	Improved dog behavior

*Exposure period 5 months.
**Interviewed 6 weeks after move.

Case History A3

Person: Son A
Age: 2½
Pre-exposure health status: Good
Health history: Term birth, normal growth and development
Previous noise exposure: No significant
Time to onset of symptoms: Immediate

	Pre-exposure	During exposure*	Post-exposure**
Sleep	Slept through night 12 hours without awakening. Always a good sleeper.	Night terrors 2–5 times each night, 30 minutes to calm down and return to quiet sleep.	At baseline. Night terrors resolved. Awakes once briefly for drink and goes back to sleep.
Headache	None	No apparent headaches.	None
Cognition	Good speech development with lots of words and no sound confusion.	Began to confuse t with k sounds and w with l sounds.	Vocabulary, sentences, and conversational skills are good but still confusing sounds.
Mood	Good-natured, sensitive, bright, listened well for age.	Oppositional, cranky, "a completely different kid for a few months."	"Instantaneous" resolution when moved, resumed former behavior.
Balance/equilibrium	Normal for age	No change	No change
Ear/hearing	Normal hearing test at birth. One episode of otitis media.	Pulled ears and got cranky synchronously with adult episodes of headache and tinnitus.	Resolved
Eye/vision	Normal	No change	No change
Other neurological	Normal	No change	No change
Cardiovascular	Normal	No change	No change
Gastrointestinal	Normal	No change	No change
Respiratory	Normal, no asthma	No change	No change

*Exposure period 5 months, age 27–32 months.
**Information provided by parents 6 weeks after move.

Case History A4

Person
Infant daughter A

Age
7 weeks

Pre-exposure health status
N/A: born 4 days before end of exposure period

Health history
Healthy newborn, 38-week gestation, birth weight 2.95 kg

Previous noise exposure
N/A

Time to onset of symptoms
N/A

	Pre-exposure	During exposure*	Post-exposure**
Sleep	In utero, 1st and 2nd trimester	In utero, 2nd and 3rd trimester	Sleeps well
Headache			N/A
Cognition			Normal alertness
Mood			Good, calms easily
Balance/equilibrium			N/A
Ear/hearing			Normal hearing test at birth
Eye/vision			Normal eye exam at birth
Other neurological	Normal fetal movement	No change	Nurses well
Cardiovascular	Normal fetal heart tones and sonogram	No change	Normal
Gastrointestinal			Normal
Respiratory			Normal

*Exposure period 5 months, all in utero.
**Information provided by parents 6 weeks after move, 7 weeks after birth.

Case History B1
(page 1 of 2)

Person
Mr. B

Age
55

Pre-exposure health status
Good

Health history
Surgery 4 times for benign prostatic hypertrophy, once for hand injury

Previous noise exposure
Diesel fishing boat from childhood

Time to onset of symptoms
Immediate with progression

	Pre-exposure	During exposure*	Post-exposure**
Sleep	Good	Delayed onset and repeated awakenings; prescribed sleep aid.	Resolved
Headache	Rare, mild	Continuous, head and ears "sizzling." "It got in your head and would dang well stay there." Started "at back of head, then down sides, then affected right eye." Prescription and non-prescription analgesics minimally helpful.	At baseline
Cognition	Normal	"Trouble remembering"; "a little problem concentrating" blamed on sleep deprivation	"Pretty good, a little problem still."
Mood	Good	Stress, "lots, pretty near more'n I could take, it just burnt me, the noise and run-around"; prescribed anxiolytic.	Improved, still takes some anxiolytic.
Balance/equilibrium	Normal, never seasick or carsick, no vertigo.	Wobbly, staggering, off-balance "like had drunk." No falls. Occasionally felt dizzy.	Resolved, on roof shingling without problems.
Ear/hearing	Normal hearing on left and mild sensorineural loss at 4 kHz on right in 2006. Intermittent left tinnitus since 2005.	Tinnitus continuous and bothersome, "ringing and sizzling," and interfering with conversation comprehension. Ears popped "like an airplane." Ear wax increased.	Resolved

Case History B1 (page 2 of 2)

	Pre-exposure	During exposure*	Post-exposure**
Eye/vision	Normal with reading glasses	Intermittent right eye pain "like a force on it, like pressure on the eye, the inside part, in the head." No change in vision. Eye pain/pressure synchronous with headache.	Resolved
Other neurological	Normal, no concussion	No change	No change
Cardiovascular	Normal with BP 126/82, 126/88, 112/70 in 2006	Mild BP elevation 140/80, 132/90, 152/92. After started anxiolytic, BP 128/84.	Resolved, BP 110/68
Gastrointestinal	Normal, no GER, not prone to nausea	Frequent nausea	Resolved
Respiratory	Slight asthma as child. Never smoked.	Two episodes of feeling of weight on chest while lying on couch, which resolved when he stood up. Lower respiratory infection in 5th month of exposure.	Normal
Rheumatologic	Osteoarthritis	No change	No change
Other	Little road traffic or other noise	"That stuff [turbine noise] doesn't get out of your head, it gets in there and just sits there—it's horrible."	Not bothered by "all kinds of traffic" at new location; "after a while you don't hear it."
		Felt pulsation in ears and chest while outside when there was fog in the valley between the turbines and the house.	Resolved
		Spent more time at shore at boat, away from house and property, for symptom relief.	
		Hum heard and felt in double glazed picture window when turbines running.	

*Exposure period 5 months.
**Interviewed 6 weeks after move.

Case History B2
(page 1 of 2)

Person
Mrs. B

Age
53

Pre-exposure health status
Good

Health history
Hysterectomy and cholecystectomy, 4 births

Previous noise exposure
Diesel fishing boat intermittently for decades

Time to onset of symptoms
Several weeks, with progression

	Pre-exposure	During exposure*	Post-exposure**
Sleep	Good	Delayed onset, repeated awakening, difficulty going back to sleep, nocturia. Ear plugs somewhat helpful.	Resolved
Headache	Rare, mild	Continuous except when left property or wind in favorable direction.	Resolved
Cognition	Normal	Concentration disturbed; confused if went on errands without list, had to return home.	Partly resolved at 6 weeks, up to remembering three things without a list.
Mood	Good, hard worker, not moody.	Anxiety, guarding against irritability, upset and "in a turmoil" when symptoms worse.	Resolved
Balance/equilibrium	Normal, never carsick or seasick.	Some unsteadiness and gait change.	Resolved
Ear/hearing	Normal hearing test in 2005, no tinnitus.	Tinnitus and ear pain continuous except when left property or wind in favorable direction. Ear irrigation at clinic worsened tinnitus.	Resolved
Eye/vision	Normal with glasses	Eyes irritated, burning, runny. Ebb and flow of eye symptoms synchronous with headache and tinnitus.	Burning resolved but visual blurring noted when chemotherapy started.
Other neurological	Normal, no concussion	No change	No change
Cardiovascular	Normal including BP	Mild BP elevations 132–140/80–90	Unknown

Case History B2 (page 2 of 2)

	Pre-exposure	During exposure*	Post-exposure**
Gastrointestinal	GER and post-tussive vomiting.	No change	Worsened with chemotherapy
Respiratory	Chronic cough secondary to GER and smoking.	Breath "short every once in a while, like [while] falling asleep, breathing wanted to catch up with something, hard to explain."	Resolved, normal breathing pattern.
Oncologic	Felt well though had undiagnosed breast cancer.	Breast cancer diagnosed. Mastectomy 4 weeks before end of exposure.	Chemotherapy started.
Other		Left house repeatedly to get relief of symptoms, interrupting work and tasks.	Resolved
Machines	Refrigerator quiet	Refrigerator became loud and was replaced, but new one was also loud.	New refrigerator was moved to new house and is quiet.
	Furnace quiet	Furnace became loud. Circulator was replaced and the furnace was still loud.	

*Exposure period 5 months.
**Interviewed 6 weeks after move.

Case History B3

	Pre-exposure	During exposure*	Post-exposure**
Sleep	Good	No change	No change
Headache	Rare, mild	No change	No change
Cognition	Good, university student	No change (between terms and not studying)	No change
Mood	"Always irritable at home"	If home more than 2 days, "heavy" feeling, lost motivation and energy, slept more	Normal energy and mood
Balance/equilibrium	Normal, never carsick or seasick	No change	No change
Ear/hearing	Ears often dry, itchy, and painful	No change	No change
Eye/vision	Normal	No change	No change
Other neurological	Normal, no concussion	No change	No change
Cardiovascular	Normal	No change	No change
Gastrointestinal	Normal	No change	No change
Respiratory	Normal, never smoked	No change	No change
Other		"Hard, heavy feeling behind ear, like someone sitting on it."	Resolved

Person
Daughter B

Age
19

Pre-exposure health status
Good

Health history
ACL tear and knee surgery

Previous noise exposure
Music

Time to onset of symptoms
Immediate

*Due to college and activities, exposure limited to 10 hours on weeknights over 2 months.
**Interviewed 7 weeks after family moved.

Case History C1 (page 1 of 2)

Person
Mr. C

Age
45

Pre-exposure health status
Good

Health history
Back injury with neuropathic pain

Previous noise exposure
Diesel fishing boat for decades

Time to onset of symptoms
Immediate when all turbines running

	Pre-exposure	During exposure*	Post-exposure**
Sleep	Good, sound sleeper	Delayed onset with repeated awakening. Wakes up tired. Feeling of pulsation keeps him awake night and day.	Improved, but not resolved because of depression.
Headache	Rare, mild	No change	No change
Cognition	Normal	Pulsations interrupt concentration; cannot read when pulsations present.	Persistent forgetfulness noted 2 years after moving, with ongoing depression.
Mood	Good	Tired, "cannot recuperate."	Persistent stress of not having his own home and loss of assets. Irritable. Enjoyed going to his abandoned home, but mood worsened with stay of several hours or more. Depression increased in winter 2 years after move.
Balance/ equilibrium	Normal, seldom seasick	No change	No change
Ear/hearing	Normal hearing, no tinnitus	Infrequent tinnitus. Hard to hear conversations outside when turbines noisy.	Resolved
Eye/vision	Normal with glasses	No change	No change
Other neurological	Normal, no concussion	No change	No change

Case History C1 (page 2 of 2)

	Pre-exposure	During exposure*	Post-exposure**
Cardiovascular	Normal including BP	No change	No change
Gastrointestinal	Normal	No change	No change
Respiratory	Normal, no smoking for 10 years	Feels pulsations in chest, holds breath, fights sensation in chest, not breathing naturally.	Resolved
Rheumatologic	Back pain from injury	No change	No change
Other		Unable to rest, relax, recuperate in house, "always in a state of defense," drives away in car to rest.	Resolved
		Feels like "energy coming within me," "like being cooked alive in a microwave."	Resolved
		Sensation of pulsation is very disturbing and interrupts concentration and sleep.	Resolved
		Infrequent sensation of throat swelling and obstruction to breathing.	Resolved
		Fog (150 days/year) amplifies noise.	
Animals		Lobster fishery moving further offshore since wind turbines present and increased death in lobster pounds.	

*Exposure period 15 months to all turbines, 21 months to at least 2 operating turbines. Interviewed 2 weeks before move and 8, 12, 18, 21, and 25 months after move.
**Ongoing partial exposure for house maintenance, increased to many hours per week during winter 2 years after moving.

Case History C2 (page 1 of 2)

Person
Mrs. C

Age
42

Pre-exposure health status
Good

Health history
Migraine disorder, 6 healthy term pregnancies without hypertension

Previous noise exposure
No significant

Time to onset of symptoms
Immediate when first turbines operational, with progression

	Pre-exposure	During exposure*	Post-exposure**
Sleep	Good	Delayed onset, frequent awakening, hyperalert when awakened, nocturia; "no good rest in 10 months."	Resolved including nocturia
Headache	Migraine frequency varied, never awoke her at night; headache onset in childhood.	Headache onset day or night, 5–6 nights/week at maximum.	Resolved, no migraines
Cognition	Normal, very organized mother of 6 children, "ready a month in advance for birthday parties."	Disorganized; could not handle as many things at once; difficult to plan and track cooking; "I thought I was half losing my mind."	Resolved including ability to multitask
Mood	Good, lots of energy	Tired, anxious, irritable.	Improved, but still sadness and stress related to loss of home and living with parents
Balance/equilibrium	Lifelong motion sensitivity in cars, boats, swings, standing on wharf seeing boats go up and down. No vertigo.	Frequent dizziness, vertigo, and nausea preceding headaches.	At baseline
Ear/hearing	Normal hearing, no tinnitus	Tinnitus began when first 2 turbines operational; no change in hearing.	Hyperacusis
Eye/vision	Normal, no glasses	Nystagmus, subjective blurring	Persistent subjective blurring
Other neurological	Normal, no concussion	No change	No change

Case History C2 (page 2 of 2)

	Pre-exposure	During exposure*	Post-exposure**
Cardiovascular	Normal including BP during pregnancies and at other times.	Hypertension and episodes of tachycardia.	Persistent BP elevation 180/102, started medications. Rare palpitations.
Gastrointestinal	Normal	Frequent nausea with dizziness and headache.	Resolved
Respiratory	Normal, never smoked	Pneumonia with pleurisy twice in first 3 months of exposure to all turbines.	Resolved
Other	Hand and foot eczema	Exacerbation	Persistent increased itching.
		At sunset, strobe effect inside or moving shadows outside triggered dizziness, nausea, and headache.	Resolved
		Occasional sensation of vibration in feet and legs outside house.	Resolved

*Exposure period 15 months to all turbines, 21 months to at least 2 operating turbines. Interviewed 2 weeks before move and 18 and 21 months after move.

**Limited ongoing exposure of several hours per week when going to house to get things, but stopped going to house by 25 months after moving.

Case History C3

Person	First son C	
Age	21	
Pre-exposure health status	Good	
Health history	Ear tubes age 13	
Previous noise exposure	Diesel fishing boat for several years	
Time to onset of symptoms	Immediate for sleep, progressive change for other symptoms	

	Pre-exposure	During exposure*	Post-exposure**
Sleep	Good	Disturbed, decreased	Resolved
Headache	Some headaches in past, frequency unclear	Frequent headaches	Resolved
Cognition	Normal, did well in elementary school, left school for fishing at age 17	Decreased concentration	No information
Mood	Angry and resistant towards parents	Very angry, never smiled, frequent and unpredictable blow-ups	Improved mood towards family and apparent increased confidence 7–8 months after move
Balance/equilibrium	Never carsick or seasick	No change	No change
Ear/hearing	Frequent otitis media in infancy/childhood; conductive hearing loss at age 13 corrected with PE tubes	Normal	No change
Eye/vision	Normal with glasses for driving only	No change	No change
Other neurological	Normal, no concussion	No change	No change
Cardiovascular	Normal including BP, one syncopal episode as teen	No change	No change
Gastrointestinal	Stomachaches as schoolchild	Normal	No change
Respiratory	Normal, no asthma or smoking	No change	No change

*Exposure period 15 months to all turbines, 21 months to at least 2 operating turbines. Out of house most of daytime for work and activities during exposure period. Information provided by parents 2 weeks before move and 8, 12, 18, and 21 months after move.

**Moved away from immediate family when family left home.

Case History C4
(page 1 of 2)

Person
Second son C

Age
19

Pre-exposure health status
Good, strong and athletic

Health history
Migraines with vomiting as older child and teen; pneumonia once; mononucleosis

Previous noise exposure
Diesel fishing boat for several years

Time to onset of symptoms
Several months

	Pre-exposure	During exposure*	Post-exposure**
Sleep	Sound sleeper with some sleep walking and talking, hard to arouse	Harder to get to sleep when he could hear turbines	Resolved
Headache	Headache with nausea and dizziness for first 2 days of each fishing trip	Occasional headache with tinnitus and dizziness on awakening	At baseline
Cognition	Normal, left school for fishing age 17; difficulty with memorization	Distracted by shadow flicker when present	Resolved
Mood	Easy-going, "jokey"	"Prickly," irritable	Resolved
Balance/equilibrium	Seasick and carsick as child with persistent symptoms on fishing trips	Occasional dizziness on awakening, as above	At baseline
Ear/hearing	Occasional tinnitus and headache from motor noise on fishing trips	Occasional tinnitus on awakening, as above	At baseline
Eye/vision	Normal, with acute peripheral and distance vision	In final month, intermittent flashes of light, then blurring, in one eye at a time at any time of day, with recovery; evolved to transient blindness (amaurosis fugax) lasting 30 seconds to 2 minutes, repetitively in each eye, right more than left; not associated with headache or tinnitus.	Persistent at 8 months and resolved at 12 months with normal vision

Case History C4 (page 2 of 2)

	Pre-exposure	During exposure*	Post-exposure**
Other neurological	Normal, one concussion as teen	After first few months, hard to move legs for first 2–5 minutes after awakening, then normal; not numb; occasional bilateral tingling around knees; knees buckled unexpectedly in daytime.	Resolved on same schedule as eye problems.
Cardiovascular	Normal including BP	No change	No change
Gastrointestinal	Normal except nausea during migraines	No change	No change
Respiratory	Normal, no asthma, smoked briefly in past	Occasionally felt pulsation in chest	Occasional difficulty taking deep breath at rest
Rheumatologic	Back injury in hockey as teen with some residual pain	Exacerbation of back pain	At baseline
Other	Hand and foot eczema	Exacerbation of eczema Slept in basement with fan on because of turbine noise	At baseline

*Exposure period 15 months to all turbines, 21 months to at least 2 operating turbines. Exposure mostly limited to nighttime in windowless basement bedroom. Interviewed 21 months after move. Information also provided by parents 2 weeks before move and 8, 12, 18, and 21 months after move.

**Moved away from immediate family when family left home.

Case History C5

Person First daughter C
Age 15
Pre-exposure health status Good
Health history No significant
Previous noise exposure No significant
Time to onset of symptoms Immediate with progression

	Pre-exposure	During exposure*	Post-exposure
Sleep	Good	Disturbed, slept better at friend's house, asked for sleeping pill	Sleeping well, no medication
Headache	Migraines, some with vomiting	Increased frequency of headache	At baseline
Cognition	Normal, good student	Mild concentration difficulty, did homework at school	Resolved
Mood	Good; compliant, shy, considerate	Marked mood swings, "PMS"	Improved
Balance/equilibrium	Normal, never carsick or seasick	Dizziness with or without headaches	Resolved
Ear/hearing	Normal	No change	No change
Eye/vision	Normal with contact lenses/glasses	No change	No change
Other neurological	Normal, no concussion	No change	No change
Cardiovascular	Normal including BP	No change	No change
Gastrointestinal	Normal	Nauseated	Resolved
Respiratory	Normal, no asthma or smoking	No change	No change

*Exposure period 15 months to all turbines, 21 months to at least 2 operating turbines. Information provided by parents 2 weeks before move and 8, 12, 18, and 21 months after move.

Case History C6

Person
Second daughter C

Age
12

Pre-exposure health status
Good

Health history
Normal growth and development

Previous noise exposure
None

Time to onset of symptoms
Immediate for sleep, 8–11 months to headache peak

	Pre-exposure	During exposure*	Post-exposure
Sleep	Good	Decreased with delayed onset	Resolved
Headache	Infrequent, moderate	Increased intensity with onset in evening 2–3 days/week, resolved with sleep, OTC analgesics sometimes helpful.	At baseline
Cognition	Good, studious, pursues activities	Completing homework at school but lost interest in schoolwork, sports, and dance lessons; "can't concentrate" per mother	Doing better in school but effort still low
Mood	Independent, active	Angry and defiant, lost friends, began smoking, suspended from school.	Improved defiance; regained "good" friends by 12 months, stopped smoking by 18 months.
Balance/equilibrium	Mildly carsick at back of van only	Occasional nausea from strobing of blades	At baseline
Ear/hearing	Normal, no tinnitus	No change	No change
Eye/vision	Normal	No change	No change
Other neurological	Normal, h/o one mild concussion	No change	No change
Cardiovascular	Normal	No change	No change
Gastrointestinal	Normal	Occasional nausea, as above	Resolved
Respiratory	Normal, no asthma	No change other than starting to smoke	No change; stopped smoking

*Exposure period 15 months to all turbines, 21 months to at least 2 operating turbines. Information provided by parents 2 weeks before move and 8, 12, 18, and 21 months after move.

Case History C7

	Pre-exposure	During exposure*	Post-exposure
Person Third son C			
Age 9			
Pre-exposure health status Good			
Health history Normal growth and development			
Previous noise exposure None			
Time to onset of symptoms Immediate for sleep, 2–5 months for schoolwork deterioration			
Sleep	Good	Decreased sleep with delayed onset	Resolved
Headache	Infrequent	Occasional, not severe	Infrequent
Cognition	Schoolwork satisfactory without need for extra help	Failed tests, lost math skills, forgot math facts. Could not maintain train of thought during homework, frustrated.	Improved but still struggling; effort less than at baseline.
Mood	Good with normal behavior	Decreased self-confidence, withdrawn behavior, fighting at school. School independently noted unexpected decline in academics and behavior.	Improved, near baseline
Balance/equilibrium	Normal, never carsick or seasick	No change	No change
Ear/hearing	Otitis media as toddler and to age 6, no rupture or tubes	Left ruptured tympanic membrane	Resolved
Eye/vision	Normal with glasses	No change	No change
Other neurological	Normal, no concussion	No change	No change
Cardiovascular	Normal	No change	No change
Gastrointestinal	Normal	No change	No change
Respiratory	Normal, no asthma	No change	No change

*Exposure period 15 months to all turbines, 21 months to at least 2 operating turbines. Information provided by parents 2 weeks before move and 8, 12, 18, and 21 months after move.

Case History C8

Person
Fourth son C

Age
5

Pre-exposure health status
Good

Health history
Normal growth and development

Previous noise exposure
None

Time to onset of symptoms
Immediate

	Pre-exposure	During exposure*	Post-exposure
Sleep	Good, to sleep at 7:30 pm	Sleep onset delayed 3 hours with many fears at night	Resolved
Headache	None	No change	No change
Cognition	Normal including school to date	"Can't concentrate" per mother	Resolved
Mood	Good with normal behavior	Angry and defiant behavior, many fears and specific fear of dying	Improved but misses 2 oldest brothers and home
Balance/equilibrium	Gets seasick and carsick	No change	No change
Ear/hearing	Normal	Complained of ears bothering him with pressure or ringing	Resolved
Eye/vision	Normal	No change	No change
Other neurological	Normal, no concussion	No change	No change
Cardiovascular	Normal	No change	No change
Gastrointestinal	Normal	No change	No change
Respiratory	Normal, no asthma	No change	No change

*Exposure period 15 months to all turbines, 21 months to at least 2 operating turbines. Information provided by parents 2 weeks before move and 8, 12, 18, and 21 months after move.

Case History D1 (page 1 of 4)

Person
Mr. D

Age
64

Pre-exposure health status
Disabled due to injury to back and neck in industrial accident, without paralysis

Health history
Ulcer age 61; current medications lovastatin, acetaminophen with codeine, laxatives

Previous noise exposure
Heavy industry age 16–37, including weaving mills, turbine and jet engine production

Time to onset of symptoms
Sleep disturbance immediate. Palpitations/tremors by 4–6 weeks. Retinal stroke at 11 weeks. Diarrhea and GI bleeding by 4 months.

	Pre-exposure	During exposure*	Post-exposure**
Sleep	No sleep problems. One acetaminophen with codeine at bedtime for back pain. Did not awaken or get up to urinate until morning.	Feels pulsation as soon as he lies down in bed. Frequent awakening, 6–12 per night. Nocturia 2–3 per night. "The worst sleep you ever heard of, up half the night." Gets to sleep using self-hypnosis he was taught for pain (counting backwards), but has to start at a higher number and count longer.	Sleeps well when away from home, without nocturia.
Headache	Rare/mild. No migraine or sinus problems.	Not headache, not painful, but a "kind of numbness which sets over the head" [see below, Balance/equilibrium]	Does not occur away from home.
Cognition	Concentration and memory good. Two-year college degree in industrial engineering.	More difficulty remembering what he reads. In last 2–3 months "I notice a little more each time." "Once I had real fast recall, but now I have to think about things."	No information
Mood	No depression, anxiety, panic, or anger problems	Frequent need to "calm down." Angry, including in night when awakened. "I can get real aggressive now and I never used to. If something doesn't go my way, I get real flustered, and then start with that nervousness and I have to go calm myself down." Irritable. Anxious about his own and wife's health and well-being.	When away for weekend, "you get all relaxed and all of a sudden you're back in the same thing again." "Getting away calms you down."

Case History D1 (page 2 of 4)

	Pre-exposure	During exposure*	Post-exposure**
Balance/ equilibrium	Never carsick but badly seasick once as a child. Avoided water ever after and disliked crossing bridges. No vertigo.	After retinal stroke, episodes of "numbness coming over my head. It seems to be my brain. Light-headed, not dizzy, I don't stagger. I can hear, I can talk, everything works for me properly, it's just that I get light-headed". No vertigo.	Does not occur away from home.
Ear/hearing	Some hearing loss but no difficulty understanding conversation. Skillfully differentiates machine noises in all settings. Has background tinnitus.	Background tinnitus is louder and higher, a "squeal" when turbines in operation. Drops in pitch when turbines are off and changes intensity when turbines change direction. When louder, the tinnitus interferes with hearing. No other sensations in ears.	Tinnitus at baseline when away from home.
Eye/vision	Wears glasses and has early cataracts.	Painless retinal stroke at night during sleep. Lost over half of vision in left eye. Confirmed by ophthalmologist, who talked to Mr. D about muscles squeezing off blood vessels in his eye. Normal CT.	No change
Other neurological	Normal without history of seizure or tremor	After 16 months: "Right arm jumps all over on its own . . . it just sits and bounces . . . hand shaking fierce just hanging onto the phone . . . started with feeling of satin or silk between the fingers . . . feels like it's wore out, like you're grabbing something real tight all the time . . . muscle spasms"; had nerve conduction studies [results unknown] and normal MRI of brain.	Arm calmed down during 5 days away and worsened on return.

Case History D1 (page 3 of 4)

	Pre-exposure	During exposure*	Post-exposure**
Cardiovascular	Normal including BP, no palpitations	Episodic tachycardia: "My heart feels like it's starting to race like crazy and I have these tremors going through my body and I was getting into a light pain on the left side of my chest." Symptoms exacerbated by nitro spray. Stress test terminated in 30 seconds. Scheduled for cardiac imaging test.	Does not occur away from home.
Gastrointestinal	Uses laxative to counteract opiate effect. Ulcer 2 years before while taking aspirin.	Stool again positive for blood; omeprazole started, endoscopy scheduled; bowels too loose or too firm.	No information
Respiratory	Normal except smoking age 15–44, no asthma	Pants or hyperventilates when tremor and tachycardia occur, and consciously slows his breathing when calming down.	Does not occur away from home.
Endocrinologic	No diabetes or other problem	No change	No change
Rheumatologic	Persistent neck and back pain due to injury at age 37. Two acetaminophen with codeine daily, rarely more. No other joint problems.	No change	No change
Other	Spent his time outside with ponies and traveled to Florida with wife for 6 weeks in winter.	"Now I don't go outside at all." At follow-up interview, the couple had not taken their next winter trip to Florida because of Mr. D's health problems.	No information
		Two months of static electric charge in yard: hair on arms would stand up when he stood in a certain area.	Static charge resolved

Case History D1 (page 4 of 4)

	Pre-exposure	During exposure*	Post-exposure**
Other (cont'd)		"When turbines get into a particular position (facing me), I get real nervous, almost like tremors going through your body . . . it's more like a vibration from outside . . . your whole body feels it, as if something was vibrating me, like sitting in a vibrating chair but my body's not moving." Occurs day or night, but not if the turbines are facing "off to the side." If outside, "I come in, sit down in my chair and try to calm myself down. After an episode like that, I'm real tired."	Does not occur away from home.
Animals	Ponies well trained for riding, jumping, and pulling cart.	Riding pony refused to leave barn, go up road, or go in field over jumps. Cart pony broke into sweats, trembled, ran uncontrolled through gates and fences with cart and harness attached. Both ponies were sold 8 weeks into exposure period.	No information
	Dog had 4 litters previously and did well.	Puppies 3 days old: mother had killed one large healthy puppy; she was staying with puppies and tolerating nursing but not licking or caring for pups.	No information

*Exposure period 6 months by first interview and 16 months at follow-up interview. Information is from first interview unless otherwise noted.
**Had purchased second house but not yet moved at follow-up interview; away only for weekends or short trips.

Case History D2
(page 1 of 2)

Person Mrs. D

Age 64

Pre-exposure health status Hypertension and cardiac output limitations

Health history 2 births and hysterectomy. Current medications: furosemide, metoprolol, felodipine, enalapril, premarin.

Previous noise exposure No significant

Time to onset of symptoms 4–5 months

	Pre-exposure	During exposure*	Post-exposure**
Sleep	Slept well	Frequent awakening	Slept well
Headache	Only at initial diagnosis of hypertension 12 years before	No change	No change
Cognition	Never was good at concentrating and did not do well in school	No change	No change
Mood	Depression with weight loss when husband injured (1983–84), treated with medication for over a year	Anger and irritability related to poor sleep; anxiety over husband's health and whether they will have to move	Improved
Balance/equilibrium	Normal, never carsick or seasick. No vertigo.	A few episodes of mild light-headedness while sitting or standing in house	Resolved
Ear/hearing	Hearing good, no tinnitus	No change	No change
Eye/vision	Normal with glasses	Having trouble reading small print at night; scheduled for eye exam	No information
Other neurological	Normal, no concussion	No change	No change
Cardiovascular	Hypertension, history of angina, history of ankle edema, limited exercise tolerance	No change	No change
Gastrointestinal	Normal	No change	No change

Case History D2 (page 2 of 2)

	Pre-exposure	During exposure*	Post-exposure**
Respiratory	Normal, no asthma or smoking	No change	No change
Endocrinologic	No diabetes	No change	No change

*Exposure period 6 months at her and her husband's first interview, 16 months at follow-up interview with husband. Information is from first interview.

**Had purchased second house but not yet moved at follow-up interview; away only for weekends or short trips.

Case History E1

Person
Mr. E

Age
56

Pre-exposure health status
Dementia, Parkinson's disease, bipolar disorder, diabetes

Health history
Hospitalized for mania three times; hospitalized at age 23 because of electric shock

Previous noise exposure
No significant

Time to onset of symptoms
Gradual

	Pre-exposure	During exposure*	Post-exposure**
Sleep	Sleep broken, "up and down all the time"	No change in pattern, but now complaining of noise and being unable to sleep	At baseline
Headache	Rare, mild	No change	No change
Cognition	No short-term memory; can't problem-solve, obsesses	No change	No change
Mood	Paranoid when manic	No change	Hypomanic after move
Balance/equilibrium	Shuffles but no overt balance problems; never carsick or seasick	Progression of Parkinsonism, decreased walking	Persistent changes
Ear/hearing	Possible decline but not tested	No change	No change
Eye/vision	Normal with glasses, no retinal changes	Blurring and retinal changes	Persistent changes
Other neurological	See Pre-exposure health status; one concussion as teen	See above	See above
Cardiovascular	Coronary artery disease, no MI, BP normal	No change	No change
Gastrointestinal	GER, constipation	No change	No change
Respiratory	Normal except smokes	No change	No change
Endocrinologic	Type II diabetes and obesity, stable on oral medication and insulin	Marked glucose instability with highs and lows	Stabilized
Other	Reduced renal function	Increased frequency of urination	Persistent changes
	Squamous cell carcinoma of skin	No new lesions	No change

*Exposure period 17 months.
**Information from interview of wife 1 month after move to new house.

Case History E2 (page 1 of 2)

Person
Mrs. E

Age
56

Pre-exposure health status
Fibromyalgia vs. reflex sympathetic dystrophy

Health history
4 term births, appendectomy, hysterectomy with "nerve damage" at age 38

Previous noise exposure
No significant

Time to onset of symptoms
Immediate with progression

	Pre-exposure	During exposure*	Post-exposure**
Sleep	Normal except after hysterectomy	Onset delayed up to 3 hours, multiple awakenings, nocturia (no glucosuria). At times awake all night, worse when blades facing NW.	Sleeps well, no nocturia
Headache	Rare, mild. Only one previous similar headache, when landing in a jet with nose and ears plugged from allergy.	Headache whenever turbines were generating, "In the wintertime, the strobing in the house and on property built up such pressure in my head you'd think it was going to blow off the top."	No headaches
Cognition	Normal: retired teacher, organizes community activities	When blades facing house, could not spell, write letters, or keep her train of thought on the telephone, but was able work when blades not facing house.	Resolved; no concentration or memory difficulties
Mood	Mild anxiety with chronic low-dose anxiolytic at bedtime	Episode of depression	At baseline
Balance/equilibrium	Never carsick or seasick. Vertigo twice in past, each episode 1–2 weeks.	"Light-headedness, head kind of swimming." Less steady on feet depending on direction blades facing, especially outside.	Resolved
Ear/hearing	Normal, tested	Occasional sensation like insect crawling in ear; no tinnitus or change in hearing	Resolved
Eye/vision	Normal, glasses for reading only	No change	No change

Case History E2 (page 2 of 2)

	Pre-exposure	During exposure*	Post-exposure**
Other neurological	Painful right leg and abdomen ascribed to nerve damage, uses TENS unit; no concussion.	Pain worse, increased use of TENS unit	Resolved when away even for short periods
Cardiovascular	Normal including BP	"Heart synchronized to rhythm of blades." When lying on back, felt "ticking" or "pulsing" in chest in rhythm with swish of the blades. Could make it stop by getting up and moving around, but started again when she lay down. Occurred more at night. No change in BP.	Resolved
Gastrointestinal	GER resolved with diet intervention.	Nauseated when she had a pounding headache.	Resolved
Respiratory	Normal, never smoked. Soprano in church choir.	More coughing illnesses, one lasting 6 weeks. Lost ability to sing.	Both resolved
Rheumatologic	Fibromyalgia; osteoarthritis in hands	Diffuse muscle aches, "thought my fibromyalgia had really flared up."	Resolved when away even for short periods
Animals	Anxious dog	Dog did not sleep, wet floor 9/10 nights	Dog dry and no longer anxious

*Exposure period 17 months.
**While away on trips of 12 days to 3 weeks and after final move 1 month before interview.

Case History F1 (page 1 of 2)

Person
Mr. F

Age
42

Pre-exposure health status
Good

Health history
No significant

Previous noise exposure
Farm equipment exposure since youth; uses hearing protection consistently

Time to onset of symptoms
3 days for sleep disturbance; 3 months for memory deficits

	Pre-exposure	During exposure*	Post-exposure**
Sleep	Rare insomnia when worried.	Frequent abrupt awakening, focusing on noise, no sleep past 4 am. Tired and "feeling beat up" in morning. Prescribed anxiolytic.	Improved, still requires occasional anxiolytic.
Headache	As teen, occipital headaches triggered by studying. No severe headaches in 20 years.	2–3 per week, not all day, increased OTC analgesic use.	1–2 per week.
Cognition	Good; BSc and registered instructor in agronomy.	Memory deficits noted from 3 months into exposure, "frustrating at times"; noise draws attention at night; concentration problems attributed to poor sleep and the lack of resolution of problem.	Concentration improved with improved sleep but memory still decreased; has ongoing depression.
Mood	Intermittent anxiety and depression since age 14, never medicated.	Depression, frustration, annoyance, anger. Unable to accomplish daily tasks.	Improved, not resolved; has more enthusiasm for doing things.
Balance/equilibrium	Slight carsickness in back seat or if reading in car. No h/o vertigo.	Occasionally off balance but not interfering with functioning.	Persists only during ongoing exposure.
Ear/hearing	"Reasonably keen hearing for age." No tinnitus.	Irritation and rumbling in ears with sensations of blowing in ears, of eardrum "moving without hearing it," and hearing noise "in center of head."	Improved with less exposure.
Eye/vision	Normal, no glasses.	No change	No change

Case History F1 (page 2 of 2)

	Pre-exposure	During exposure*	Post-exposure**
Other neurological	Normal, no concussion.	No change	No change
Cardiovascular	Infrequent tachycardia of short duration (5 seconds), diagnosed at age 15.	Weekly episodes of tachycardia of increased duration, longest 15 minutes.	Frequency still increased
Gastrointestinal	Intermittent GER and irritable bowel symptoms.	Increased frequency and intensity of GER and irritable bowel symptoms.	Unresolved
Respiratory	Mild wheezing with URIs began about 6 years before, no medication prescribed.	Pneumonia and asthma diagnosed 6 weeks into exposure; thereafter, persistent wheezing requiring use of bronchodilator about twice a week.	Persistent opacity on chest x-ray and semiweekly wheezing
Rheumatologic	Intermittent knee arthralgia since age 11 related to overuse.	No change	No change
Other		Detected indoor vibration/hum more after double-glazed windows installed in attempt to exclude noise.	

*Exposure period 7 months until rented "sleeping house" and 12 months until rented "sleeping and living house."
**Ongoing exposure up to 8 hours per day while farming land and using farm office in home. Interviewed 3 months after second exposure reduction.

Case History F2 (page 1 of 2)

Person
Mrs. F

Age
51

Pre-exposure health status
Good with controlled asthma

Health history
Breast cancer with mastectomy 2002; preeclampsia 1990; 2 births; current medications anastrazol, beclamethasone inhaler, salmeterol inhaler

Previous noise exposure
No significant

Time to onset of symptoms
3 days

	Pre-exposure	During exposure*	Post-exposure**
Sleep	Good	3–6 hours of disrupted sleep/night. Startles awake with heart pounding, feeling of fear, compulsion to check house, and need to urinate, then unable to go back to sleep. Tired in morning. Prescribed anxiolytic.	Normal sleep without medication on any night away
Headache	Rare, mild	Daily, long-lasting, with increased OTC analgesic use. Headaches worse with consecutive days of exposure.	Resolved with reduced exposure
Cognition	Good, master's level nurse, midwife, and health administrator	Could not follow recipes, plots of TV shows, or furniture assembly instructions.	Improved, not resolved
Mood	Normal	Depression, despair, hopelessness, exhaustion, "feeling of unease all the time" and of being overwhelmed.	Improved, not resolved
Balance/equilibrium	Occasional motion sickness on boat or carnival ride. No h/o vertigo.	Frequent nausea with occasional dizzy feeling.	Resolved except with prolonged or overnight exposure
Ear/hearing	High frequency hearing loss due to chemotherapy. No tinnitus. No h/o otitis media.	Prolonged (3 week) first-time otitis media. No tinnitus, no change in hearing.	At baseline
Eye/vision	Normal with glasses	Mild blurring in one eye some mornings.	Improved

Case History F2 (page 2 of 2)

	Pre-exposure	During exposure*	Post-exposure**
Other neurological	Normal, no concussion	No change	No change
Cardiovascular	Occasional palpitations. BP 130/80 range, stable x 17 years	Palpitations unchanged, BP increasing during exposure period.	BP 150/90–108; started antihypertensive
Gastrointestinal	Intermittent mild GER not requiring medication	Began treatment with proton pump inhibitor; nauseated if sleeps in home or spends longer hours there.	No nausea or need for proton pump inhibitor
Respiratory	Well-controlled asthma	No change	No change
Other		Physical sensation of noise "like a heavy rock concert."	
		"Hum makes you feel sick."	
		"We are talking about the complete devastation of your life."	
		Visiting adult son, 10 pm: "We're going to go stay in a nightclub. It would be quieter."	
Animals	Moles throughout lawn	No moles	Molehill appears when turbines off for 3–4 days.
	Dog slept in outdoor kennel.	Dog refuses to sleep in kennel, sleeps only in garage next to freezer, and barks to get in.	Dog's behavior persistent even when turbines off.

*Exposure period 7 months until rented "sleeping house" and 12 months until rented "sleeping and living house."
**Ongoing exposure up to 8 hours per day while farming land and using farm office in home. Interviewed 3 months after second exposure reduction.

Case History F3 (page 1 of 2)

Person
Daughter F

Age
17

Pre-exposure health status
Good

Health history
Frequent otitis media as child, no PE tubes; intermittent mild asthma

Previous noise exposure
No significant: plays grand piano, keeps iPod volume and bass low

Time to onset of symptoms
Noticed gradually, especially by contrast after family vacation

	Pre-exposure	During exposure*	Post-exposure**
Sleep	Good	Poor sleep, not rested in morning, began taking naps after school	Sleeps well in sleeping house, not tired in day
Headache	Rare, mild	Increased, with increased OTC analgesic use	Resolved
Cognition	Good. Studies and reading require diligent effort. High marks on GCSE national exams at age 16.	Marks on AS national exams at age 17 were significantly lower than past performance and school expectations. Regular school marks and tests in usual range.	Improved
Mood	Good, conscientious	Irritable, argumentative, unwilling to do things, "more depressed than usual for teenagers," she stated	Annoyed at having to travel to sleep
Balance/equilibrium	Normal, never carsick or seasick	No change	No change
Ear/hearing	Normal hearing	No change	No change
Eye/vision	Normal with small correction for reading	Persistent floater in one eye, examined by optometrist	No change
Other neurological	Normal, no concussion	No change	No change
Cardiovascular	Normal including BP	No change	No change
Gastrointestinal	Normal	No change	No change

Case History F3 (page 2 of 2)

	Pre-exposure	During exposure*	Post-exposure**
Respiratory	Mild asthma only with URIs. No bronchodilator use in 2 years before exposure.	Daily bronchodilator use began at 6 months; two prolonged lower respiratory infections at 7 and 8 months; low peak flows persisted 3 months after infections, when inhaled steroid added.	Continuing inhaled steroid use, peak flows resolved
Other		Did not hear or feel anything except "whooshing" some nights.	

*Exposure period 7 months until rented "sleeping house" and 12 months until rented "sleeping and living house."
**Limited ongoing exposure after school and on weekends/vacations. Interviewed 3 months after second exposure reduction.

Case History F4
(page 1 of 2)

Person
Mrs. F Senior

Age
75

Pre-exposure health status
Atrial fibrillation, anticoagulation, memory loss

Health history
Colostomy 1989 for obstruction, reversed 1991; current medications warfarin, digoxin

Previous noise exposure
No significant

Time of onset of symptoms
Immediate with progression

	Pre-exposure	During exposure*	Post-exposure**
Sleep	Satisfactory, no daytime naps; one void nightly with brief awakening	Awakened 2–3 times per night when wind from direction of turbines; feels "very awake, not relaxed" when awakened; prolonged nighttime awake periods. Nocturia with urge to void at each awakening. Taking daytime naps.	Slept well in hospital at 18 months' exposure, otherwise has not left home
Headache	Rare, mild	No change	
Cognition	Mild memory and cognitive abnormalities	No change	
Mood	Good as long as she can go out in her garden	No change, still going outside	
Balance/equilibrium	Normal, never carsick or seasick, no h/o vertigo	No change	
Ear/hearing	Hearing satisfactory	"I can feel it in my ears" at times of night awakenings; feels like "wax or someone blowing down your ears."	
Eye/vision	Normal with glasses	No change	
Other neurological	Normal, no concussion	No change	
Cardiovascular	Atrial fibrillation with anticoagulation x 10 years, stable on 2–4 mcg warfarin daily	INR decreased and warfarin dose increased to 8–9 mcg daily; at 18 months acute exacerbation of AF during pneumonia/pyelonephritis.	

Case History F4 (page 2 of 2)

	Pre-exposure	During exposure*	Post-exposure**
Gastrointestinal	Normal functioning, asymptomatic	No change	
Respiratory	Normal, no asthma, never smoked	Persistent "bad cough" for 3–4 months starting at 8 months; took antibiotic, cough improved, then recurred. Pneumonia with hypoxia at 18 months followed by persistent dyspnea; at 20 months, scarring on chest CT at both lung apices and site of pneumonia; under investigation by pulmonologist.	
Rheumatologic	No arthritis	Onset of arthritis in one knee; acute swelling at 18 months yielded no fluid; under investigation by rheumatologist.	
Renal	Normal	Nocturia; pyelonephritis at 18 months	
Animals	Dog went outside and in various rooms in house.	Dog stays in kitchen.	

*Interviewed at 16 months of exposure; health updates provided by daughter-in-law to 21 months of exposure. Information from interview unless otherwise noted.

**Mrs. F Senior did not reduce her exposure with her son and his family.

Case History G1 (page 1 of 2)

Person
Mr. G

Age
32

Pre-exposure health status
Good

Health history
Chronic bilateral serous otitis media and conductive hearing loss treated with PE tubes at ages 7 and 9

Previous noise exposure
Ongoing exposure to airplane and train noise while commuting

Time to onset of symptoms
Noticed gradually

	Pre-exposure	During exposure*	Post-exposure
Sleep	Good	Delayed onset and increased awakening due to noise. Uses ear plugs.	Not disturbed by urban rail line outside window during work week. Slept well when away with family and after move.
Headache	A few bad headaches in life, not identified as migraines	If awakened by turbine noise, has headache at time of awakening and in morning	No headaches
Cognition	Good; computer programmer; long work days and commute	Tired at work, "concentration lacking in afternoons"	At baseline with same commute; tired but concentration fine
Mood	Good	Finds noise outside or noise which awakens him at night stressful. Worried about wife and family.	Feels more relaxed; situation resolved; wife and children all happier; home with family every day.
Balance/ equilibrium	Always seasick; carsick if in back seat. Vertigo for a few weeks at age 29.	Episodes of dizziness "like being spun fast in a circle"; disorientation/feeling "very strange" in certain parts of house at certain times where he can "feel rumbling."	Did not occur away from exposed home, when turbines off, or after moving
Ear/hearing	Normal hearing; no tinnitus	No change	No change
Eye/vision	Corrected with glasses; eyestrain from computer work	No change	No change

Case History G1 (page 2 of 2)

	Pre-exposure	During exposure*	Post-exposure
Other neurological	Normal, no concussion	No change	No change
Cardiovascular	Normal including BP	No symptoms, BP not measured	No change
Gastrointestinal	Normal	Moves away from spot in house where he feels strange before it progresses to nausea.	Did not occur away from exposed home, when turbines off, or after moving.
Respiratory	Slight asthma with dust/mold allergies, intermittent bronchodilator use. Never smoked.	No change	No change
Other		"Noise at times is very invasive. Train noise has a different quality, not invasive." "Flicker is visually invasive."	

*During 15 month exposure, exposure reduced by working and staying in a distant city Mon–Fri each week; at home weekends; traveled by plane and train. Interviewed after 11 months of exposure and 2 months after moving away.

Case History G2 (page 1 of 3)

Person Mrs. G

Age 32

Pre-exposure health status Good

Health history Episode of depression at age 18; 4 births, no post-partum depression

Previous noise exposure No significant

Time to onset of symptoms 3 months for concentration problem, 10 months for depression (when infant 7 months old)

	Pre-exposure	During exposure*	Post-exposure
Sleep	Good	Sleep onset delayed up to 4 hours; turbine noise wakes up children, 2-year-old with night terrors/ screaming; tired in morning.	Goes to sleep quickly; children sleep through night; well-rested; not bothered by traffic noise; immediate resolution.
Headache	Migraine with aura once a year	Migraine frequency increased to 4/year; also prolonged, "heavy" frontal headaches and "a permanent fuzz in my head."	Frontal headaches resolved immediately; no migraines since move; one mild headache every few weeks which resolves quickly on its own.
Cognition	Normal, well organized; no cognitive deficits even with previous depression	Forgetful, has to write everything down, can't seem to get organized, hard to concentrate	Concentration and memory gradually improving; she rated them 10/10 pre-exposure, 2/10 during exposure, and 5/10 2 months after moving.
Mood	Good (see Health history)	Irritable, angry, worried about future and children, developing depression; better when turbines off and can go outside.	Improved, regaining energy, "bouncing around again," enjoying children. She rated her mood 10/10 before exposure, 2/10 during exposure, and 7/10 2 months after moving.

Case History G2 (page 2 of 3)

	Pre-exposure	During exposure*	Post-exposure
Balance/equilibrium	Slight carsickness even as adult; seasick only when pregnant. No h/o vertigo.	Disoriented, "light-headed," dizzy, and nauseated in garden and specific parts of house where she detects vibration; feels her body is vibrating "inside" but walls, windows, and objects are not vibrating. No balance problem.	Did not occur away from exposed home, when turbines off, or after moving
Ear/hearing	Good, no tinnitus	Hyperacusis; finds TV unbearably loud.	Resolved, hearing sensitivity at baseline
Eye/vision	Normal with glasses	No change	No change
Other neurological	Normal, no concussion	No change	No change
Cardiovascular	Normal except BP increase during 3rd and 4th pregnancies	No symptoms, BP not checked	No change
Gastrointestinal	Normal, no GER	Nauseated; see Balance/equilibrium	Resolved
Respiratory	Mild asthma, no inhaler use in 7 years	No change; normal coughs and colds from children	Same; new colds in new location
Rheumatologic	No joint problems	Sharp pain in elbow on lifting	Resolved when away from exposed home for 1–3 weeks and recurred upon return; resolved immediately when moved, despite increased lifting during move.
Other		Noise similar to a diesel tractor-trailer on other side of house wall	Traffic noise at new home on busy road is not bothersome, especially because it slacks off at night
		Can hear turbines over a 90-dB lawnmower because of quality of noise	

Case History G2 (page 3 of 3)

	Pre-exposure	During exposure*	Post-exposure
Animals	Bats lived in unused chimney; family did not disturb them	Bats gone	
	Three deer seen regularly in yard and many others in neighborhood	Deer no longer present, moved downhill to village	
	Dogs quiet at night	Dogs bark a lot at night	

*Exposure period 15 months. Interviewed after 11 months of exposure and 2 months after moving away.

Case History G3 (page 1 of 2)

Person
First son G

Age
6 (7 post-exposure)

Pre-exposure health status
Normal growth/development

Health history
No significant

Previous noise exposure
No significant

Time to onset of symptoms
Immediate with progression

	Pre-exposure	During exposure*	Post-exposure
Sleep	Sleeps through night	Appeared to sleep through night but frequently told mother in morning he was "sitting up all night"; felt tired and looked "permanently tired."	Not claiming to "sit up all night," doesn't look as tired.
Headache	No headaches	Headaches when he plays video games and when he hasn't played them for days	Still plays video games but no headaches.
Cognition	Extremely focused child, advanced in reading	Never liked to read on own or a whole book	Sits down to read on his own for an hour at a time and reads "quite a thick book."
Mood	Normal	"Freaked out" over going to store with mother and siblings, tantrums and bad moods prolonged.	Happier, less grouchy, gets over his resistance and tantrums quickly.
Balance/equilibrium	Gets carsick and seasick	No change	No change
Ear/hearing	Chronic serous otitis media in one ear with reduced hearing	Persistent	Persistent
Eye/vision	Normal	No change	No change
Other neurological	Normal, no concussion	No change	No change
Cardiovascular	Normal	No change	No change

Case History G3 (page 2 of 2)

	Pre-exposure	During exposure*	Post-exposure
Gastrointestinal	Normal	No change	No change
Respiratory	Normal, no asthma	No change	No change
Other		Less time outdoors because of turbine noise	

*Exposure period 15 months. Information provided by parents after 11 months of exposure and 2 months after moving away.

Case History G4
(page 1 of 2)

Person
First daughter G

Age
5

Pre-exposure health status
Normal growth/development

Health history
Repetitive otitis media with bilateral chronic serous otitis media, no PE tubes

Previous noise exposure
No significant

Time to onset of symptoms
Immediate with progression

	Pre-exposure	During exposure*	Post-exposure
Sleep	Slept through night	Awakened by turbine noise, saying, "I can hear this horrible noise." Could be soothed by mother and return to sleep. Wet bed half of nights, 2–3 nights in a row.	Sleeps through night. No bed-wetting while away from exposed home for 1–3 week visits or since move.
Headache	None	No change	No change
Cognition	Normal, no teacher concerns, but mother notes short attention span.	Hearing loss thought to be affecting school work.	Hearing and ear fluid unchanged, but "schoolwork has improved massively."
Mood	Normal for age	Tantrums over homework only: "I can't do it, I can't do it," then storming out of room.	More patient and can work longer on homework.
Balance/ equilibrium	Never carsick or seasick, balance good	No change	No change
Ear/hearing	Bilateral conductive hearing loss due to middle ear fluid	Persistent throughout exposure period with bilateral hearing loss and frequent episodes of acute otitis media	No change from exposure period, on waiting list for PE tubes
Eye/vision	Normal	No change	No change
Other neurological	Normal, no concussion	No change	No change
Cardiovascular	Normal	No change	No change
Gastrointestinal	Normal	No change	No change

Case History G4 (page 2 of 2)

	Pre-exposure	During exposure*	Post-exposure
Respiratory	Normal, no asthma	No change	No change
Other		Less time outdoors because of turbine noise	

*Exposure period 15 months. Information provided by parents after 11 months of exposure and 2 months after moving away.

Case History G5
(page 1 of 2)

Person
Second daughter G

Age
2 (at both interviews)

Pre-exposure health status
Normal growth/development

Health history
Eczema as baby

Previous noise exposure
No significant

Time to onset of symptoms
Immediate with progression

	Pre-exposure	During exposure*	Post-exposure
Sleep	Sleeps through night	Whenever turbines noisy, awakened screaming, climbing out of bed; easily comforted by mom but grabbed posts to resist going back in own bed; had to sleep with mom.	Rarely awakens at night, no screaming, okay to go back into own bed after little cuddle.
Headache	None	Did not hold head, but spent some days quietly on couch after receiving OTC analgesic.	Never spends day on couch; energetic even with URI.
Cognition	Normal development	Good language development	Good language development
Mood	Normal	Irritable, oversensitive; numerous crying/screaming bouts every day if a sibling "unsteadied her or even walked too close."	Bouncy, good-natured, confident, "gives as good as she gets" and doesn't melt down or overreact.
Balance/equilibrium	Never carsick or seasick	No change	No change
Ear/hearing	Normal, no h/o otitis media	No otitis media even with URIs	No change
Eye/vision	Normal	No change	No change
Other neurological	Normal, no concussion	No change	No change
Cardiovascular	Normal	No change	No change
Gastrointestinal	Normal	No change	No change

Case History G5 (page 2 of 2)

	Pre-exposure	During exposure*	Post-exposure
Respiratory	Normal, no asthma	No change	No change
Other		Less time outdoors because of turbine noise	

*Exposure period 15 months. Information provided by parents after 11 months of exposure and 2 months after moving away.

Case History G6

	Pre-exposure	During exposure*	Post-exposure
Person Infant son G			
Age 8 months (14 months at 2nd interview)			
Pre-exposure health status Term healthy infant exposed final 3 months in utero			
Health history Slight eczema			
Previous noise exposure No significant			
Time to onset of symptoms No symptoms			
Sleep	N/A	Slept through night from 6 weeks of age	Continues to sleep through night
Headache		N/A	N/A
Cognition		No developmental concerns	At 14 months, "Not the quiet one in the corner anymore—starting to chat now, making the right noises." Pulling up and cruising around furniture, very sociable.
Mood		"Always a very laid-back little boy"	No change
Balance/equilibrium		N/A	At 14 months, not yet walking independently
Ear/hearing		Normal	No change
Eye/vision		Normal	No change
Other neurological	Normal fetal movement	Normal	No change
Cardiovascular	Normal fetal heart tones and sonogram	Normal	No change
Gastrointestinal		Normal	No change
Respiratory		Normal	No change

*Exposure period 15 months, 3 months in utero and 12 months as infant. Information provided by parents when he was 8 months old and 2 months after moving away.

Case History H1

Person Mr. H
Age 52
Pre-exposure health status Good
Health history No significant other than PTSD
Previous noise exposure Served in army; drives buses and milk tanker truck
Time to onset of symptoms Immediate for sleep disturbance

	Pre-exposure	During exposure*	Post-exposure**
Sleep	Good; not disturbed by traffic/train noise at former home	Awakened by turbine noise 2–3 times a week, tired next day	Sleeps through night, better rested
Headache	Rare headache	No change	No change
Cognition	Memory problems since event which caused PTSD, forgets experiences and things to do until reminded	No change	No change
Mood	PTSD/depression 4 years before exposure	No exacerbation	No change
Balance/equilibrium	Never carsick or seasick, no h/o vertigo	No change	No change
Ear/hearing	"Near perfect" hearing, no tinnitus	Mild continuous "static noise" tinnitus, not affecting hearing	Unknown
Eye/vision	Normal with glasses	No change	No change
Other neurological	Normal, mild concussion age 39	No change	No change
Cardiovascular	Normal including BP	No change	No change
Gastrointestinal	Normal, occasional diarrhea	No change	No change
Respiratory	Normal except smokes	No change	No change
Rheumatologic	No joint problems	Arthritis in one finger joint	Unknown

*Exposure period 2 years; away from house 3 am to 4–5 pm daily for work.
**Family has not moved but was away from home for 2 weeks in the 2 months preceding the interview.

Case History H2 (page 1 of 2)

Person
Mrs. H

Age
57

Pre-exposure health status
Lupus with arthritis and normal renal function; takes quinine; also diagnosed with fibromyalgia

Health history
Hysterectomy and lipoma removal

Previous noise exposure
Urban life to age 54

Time to onset of symptoms
Immediate with progression

	Pre-exposure	During exposure*	Post-exposure**
Sleep	Slept well through night	Delayed onset and frequent awakening, 5–6 per night; awakens with sense of fear, compulsion to check house, "very disturbed sort of waking up, you jolt awake, like someone has broken a pane of glass to get into the house; you know what it is but you've got to check it—go open the front door—it's horrific"; nocturia; unable to go back to sleep	Slept well through night
Headache	Rare, mild	Headaches continuous unless turbines off; takes analgesics only when headache very bad in night.	No headaches while away
Cognition	Concentration/memory problems when first diagnosed with lupus, then improved	Concentration/memory slightly worse, writing herself more reminders	At pre-exposure baseline
Mood	No h/o mood problem or anxiety	Irritable and angry, shouting more	Improved while away
Balance/equilibrium	Never carsick or seasick; 4 episodes of vertigo, all 6 or more years before exposure	10–20 minute episodes of dizziness, sometimes with nausea	Did not occur while away
Ear/hearing	Tinnitus and hearing loss	Ongoing tinnitus and 3 incidents, each 1 hour at 3–4 am, of "real high-pitched noise, holding my head, not in ears, just in head, not something I could hear." Also intermittent ear pain, "not earache."	Did not occur while away

Case History H2 (page 2 of 2)

	Pre-exposure	During exposure*	Post-exposure**
Eye/vision	Diplopia requiring prisms in glasses began at least 6 years before exposure	Intermittent blurring (can't read letters on TV) and dry, sore feeling in eyes	Unknown
Other neurological	Diplopia; concussion around beginning of exposure period	No change	No change
Cardiovascular	Normal including BP	No change	No change
Gastrointestinal	Normal	Repetitive belching with feeling of air trapping and soreness of chest wall; rubs chest, lies on side to release air and obtain relief.	Unknown
Respiratory	Short of breath around polish or perfumes; feather allergy; smokes	No change	No change
Rheumatologic	Joint and muscle pains, not exacerbated by weather	Pain worse and continuous. Began with exacerbation of muscle and joint pains, then neck pain and headaches; when returned from trip, pain built back up over a week.	Improved to baseline level
Other	No problem with noise from truck traffic or living in flight path of small airport	Turbine noise different, "unnatural"; sounds like airplane stuck over house; pulsation prevents sleep; sound intensifies in cold weather.	"When I'm away it's so different, it's like I'm in a normal life."
	Cottage heated by two open coal fires	Both chimneys taken down and roof replaced, with extra insulation, in attempt to keep noise out; coal fires replaced by electric oil-filled radiators; cottage became damper.	

*Exposure period 2 years; family lived here 1 year before turbines went into operation.
**Family has not moved but was away from home for 2 weeks in the 2 months preceding the interview.

Case History H3

Person
Grandson H

Age
8

Pre-exposure health status
Healthy with normal development

Health history
No significant

Previous noise exposure
No significant

Time to onset of symptoms
Immediate for sleep, gradual for mood and concentration

	Pre-exposure	During exposure*	Post-exposure**
Sleep	Slept quietly through night	Difficulty falling asleep, irritable at bedtime. When asleep, kicking and moving all night. In bed 11 hours/night.	Slept well
Headache	Rare	Increased but still infrequent	No headache
Cognition	Does well in reading, spelling, and math; excellent memory.	Teacher told him he was not concentrating and needed to go to bed earlier; resistant to doing homework.	Not in school while away
Mood	Calm, intelligent child with good language abilities	Irritable, tired, lethargic, aggressive; shouts, stamps, refuses.	Improved while away
Balance/equilibrium	Normal, never carsick	No change	No change
Ear/hearing	Normal, no h/o otitis media	No change	No change
Eye/vision	Poor vision (shapes only) in left eye; right has normal acuity	Started to "squint", eye exam pending.	No change
Other neurological	Normal, no concussion	No change	No change
Cardiovascular	Normal	No change	No change
Gastrointestinal	Normal	No change	No change
Respiratory	Normal, no asthma	No change	No change

*Exposure period two years; away from home at school 6 hours per day during school year.
**Family has not moved but was away from home for 2 weeks in the 2 months preceding the interview.

Case History I1 (page 1 of 2)

Person
Mr. I

Age
59

Pre-exposure health status
Healthy, active

Health history
No significant

Previous noise exposure
Church bell ringer as child; lawn mowers, chain saws as gardener, mostly with hearing protection

Time to onset of symptoms
2 months

	Pre-exposure	During exposure*	Post-exposure**
Sleep	Slept well	One long awakening each noisy night	
Headache	None	No change	
Cognition	Normal, no concentration or memory problems	Cannot concentrate on his outdoor gardening and building tasks; "after half an hour you have to leave, escape, close the door."	
Mood	Happy	Anger, anxiety, depression, feeling of shame and powerlessness; well motivated to work for others but not outside in own garden	
Balance/equilibrium	Never carsick or seasick, no h/o vertigo	No change	
Ear/hearing	Difficulty following conversation in loud restaurant; no tinnitus	Tinnitus "like waterfall noise"	
Eye/vision	Normal with glasses	No change	
Other neurological	Normal, mild concussion age 9	No change	
Cardiovascular	Normal including BP	No change	

Case History I1 (page 2 of 2)

	Pre-exposure	During exposure*	Post-exposure**
Gastrointestinal	Normal	Ill-defined problem with digestion in the morning, long-term; noise at times "so irritating I want to be sick."	
Respiratory	Normal	No change	
Other	"My wife had a small firm; as a gardener I had enough money."	"All we had saved is gone [went into new house]; no one will buy our house."	

*Interviewed after 13 months of ongoing exposure.
**Has not gone away for a prolonged period or moved.

Case History 12 (page 1 of 3)

Person
Mrs. I

Age
52

Pre-exposure health status
Excellent with minor back pain

Health history
Tonsillectomy age 24, hysterectomy age 39, 3 births

Previous noise exposure
Grew up near major urban airport

Time to onset of symptoms
2 months

	Pre-exposure	During exposure*	Post-exposure**
Sleep	Normal with culturally appropriate nap in summer	1–3 awakenings on noisy nights after 4 hours of sleep, weeping in night; "When I wake up, more a feeling of pressure and tightness in chest; it makes me panic and feel afraid"; "a startling sort of waking up, a feeling there was something and I don't know what it was"; feelings of panic keep her from going back to sleep; once woke thinking there had been an earth tremor (there had not); no delay getting to sleep or nocturia; tired only after wakeful night	Slept well
Headache	No headaches	"Not excruciating" or major problem; pressure in front, sides, back; rare aspirin	No headaches
Cognition	Good, master's level multilingual teacher, ran own business	No change in concentration or memory	No change
Mood	Depression 3 months at age 19 and brief postpartum depression with first baby only; "usually cheerful nature"	Anxiety, foreboding, and anger evolving to depression; "strong mental and physical agitation"; takes pains not to be irritable; frequent unexpected crying; despairing of future; consulted psychiatrist	Resolved, felt normal, no depression. When returned home, "immediately struck by uncontrollable bouts of crying"

Case History 12 (page 2 of 3)

	Pre-exposure	During exposure*	Post-exposure**
Balance/equilibrium	Very carsick as child, still carsick as passenger and seasick; no h/o vertigo	No change; no dizziness or balance disturbance	No change
Ear/hearing	Hearing normal, no tinnitus	Episodic bilateral sensation of "pressure in my ears and sometimes ringing" and sometimes pain; "feeling the vibration is in my head, behind my ear drums, somewhere inside, very local" or "around the canal that leads to the ear drum"; tinnitus noticeable but not loud, low to medium pitch, does not interfere with understanding conversation; 2–3 episodes per week, including on awakening at night	Resolves after half a day when leaves or turbines completely silent and still
Eye/vision	Normal with glasses	No change	No change
Other neurological	Normal, no concussion	Episodic "trembling in arms, legs, fingers"	No change
Cardiovascular	Normal including BP	Twice awoke with palpitations, "feeling your heart is beating very fast and very loud, so I can feel the blood pumping"; no change in BP	Resolved
Gastrointestinal	Normal	Episodic "queasiness and nausea," loss of appetite	Resolved
Respiratory	Normal, smoked age 15–25, then none to once a month	Vibratory feeling mostly in chest, feels like "pins and needles"; chest tightness on awakening at night	Resolved

Case History 12 (page 3 of 3)

	Pre-exposure	During exposure*	Post-exposure**
Rheumatologic	Mild back pain	No change	No change
Other		Noise inside house "low, pulsating, almost a vibration" not shut out by earplugs; "It affects my body; this is the feeling I get when I say I'm agitated or jittery. It's this that gives me pressure or ringing in my ears"	Resolved
		"A feeling someone has invaded not only my health and my territory, but my body"	Resolved
Animals	Bees swarm in spring; locally, other bee problems before turbines	Repetitive, chaotic swarming through summer	

*Exposure 10 months, left home for 10 weeks, back home for 2 weeks at time of interview. Provided journal maintained throughout exposure period.
**During 10 weeks away from home.

Case History J1
(page 1 of 2)

Person
Dr. J

Age
49

Pre-exposure health status
Good

Health history
Broken nose repair as teen; thyroglossal duct cyst excision as child

Previous noise exposure
Uses tractors and chain saws on property with hearing protection

Time to onset of symptoms
Immediate with progression

	Pre-exposure	During exposure*	Post-exposure**
Sleep	Long-term difficulty with returning to sleep started during medical training, had been improving	Delayed sleep onset and frequent awakening when turbines running fast; awakens with racing heart; can't get back to sleep; taking prescription sleep aid	Improved sleep, no need for sleep aid
Headache	Infrequent sinus headache, no migraines	Bilateral temporo-parietal headaches 3–4 times a week; may follow a "jittery" episode	No headaches
Cognition	Good; specialist physician	Difficulty with focus and mental energy after nights of poor sleep; marked concentration problem when doing accounts/bills at home	Concentration seemed fine but demand low
Mood	Good, no history of anxiety or depression	"Jittery" episodes begin with sensation of "internal quivering" or awakening with rapid or pounding heart; gets "real anxious"; has to stop outdoor or family activities and go indoors; at night has to move to basement where the turbines cannot be heard or felt; on arriving home from work, he can judge from the rotational speed of the turbines or the noise and feeling of vibration in the garage whether symptoms will be triggered; increased irritability; taking two anti-anxiety medications	No "jittery" episodes or anxiety when away or at work; no need for anxiolytic

Case History J1 (page 2 of 2)

	Pre-exposure	During exposure*	Post-exposure**
Balance/equilibrium	Good, seasick once in life	3 episodes of transient vertigo/dizziness while in tree stands late in day	No dizziness or vertigo
Ear/hearing	Slight left hearing loss on test 10 years prior; tinnitus during sinus infections	No subjective change in hearing; occasional tinnitus outdoors when turbines spinning rapidly	At baseline; no tinnitus
Eye/vision	Normal with glasses	Developing presbyopia (expected for age)	No change
Other neurological	Normal with mild concussion age 7	No change	No change
Cardiovascular	Normal including BP; no palpitations	BP normal but not measured during "jittery" episodes; awakens with rapid or pounding heart and "jittery" sensations when turbines noisy.	No "jittery" episodes
Gastrointestinal	Normal without GER or nausea	Queasiness and reduced appetite in evening with onset as he arrives home from work	No nausea, appetite good
Respiratory	Normal without asthma; smoked age 18–23	No change	No change
Other	Farming, building, and hunting activities for relaxation at home	Home more stressful than work; driven inside from farming activities, picnics, playing with sons, and hunting by turbine noise provoking symptomatic episodes.	Able to relax outdoors
Animals		Horse, 5 beef cattle, ducks unaffected	

*Interviewed after 9 months of exposure. Family has not moved.
**Away for vacation for 2 weeks during the first 3 months of exposure and 10 days during the month before the interview.

Case History J2 (page 1 of 2)

Person
Mrs. J

Age
47

Pre-exposure health status
Good

Health history
2 term births

Previous noise exposure
Aircraft during medical evacuations

Time to onset of symptoms
1–3 months to headaches;
1–3 months to concentration and memory problems;
4–5 months to continuous palpitations;
6 months to exacerbation of irritable bowel

	Pre-exposure	During exposure*	Post-exposure**
Sleep	Slept well under any circumstances	Falls asleep easily; if awakened, can usually go back to sleep	Slept well
Headache	No headaches	Evening headache at least every 2 weeks requiring ibuprofen	No headaches
Cognition	Good; acute/critical care nurse; teaches nursing at university; organized mother; no problem with focus or memory	Noticeable trouble focusing and remembering at home; has to write down what children tell her or any item to be picked up at store; easily distracted; started vitamins and supplements	Memory improved when away but not to baseline (also less demand)
Mood	Happy, energetic, busy, "up" person	Marked decrease in energy and motivation at home; frustrated; "on edge"; feels rejuvenated at work	Felt great, lots of energy
Balance/ equilibrium	Never carsick or seasick, no h/o vertigo	No change	No change
Ear/hearing	Normal, tested yearly; no tinnitus	No change, no ear symptoms	No change
Eye/vision	Normal, wears contact lenses	No change	No change
Other neurological	Normal, no concussion	No change	No change

Case History J2 (page 2 of 2)

	Pre-exposure	During exposure*	Post-exposure**
Cardiovascular	Normal BP except during first pregnancy; dysrhythmia (trigeminy) 10/06 resolved with caffeine restriction	Continuous palpitations began 10/07 and did not respond to caffeine restriction or trials of two medications; evaluated including electrophysiology; right ventricular focus	Decreased frequency of palpitations
Gastrointestinal	Irritable bowel (cramping and diarrhea) since young adulthood with exacerbations before exams; normal colonoscopy x 2	Continuous symptoms for 3 months before interview, except during week after return from vacation	Symptoms unchanged while away in tropical country
Respiratory	Normal, no asthma, never smoked	No change	No change
Other		Feels vibration in feet/lower legs when stands still in house or barn, which feels like it is coming from vibrations in the structure; worse in barn, which is not insulated; does not feel this outside/on the ground Sounds like helicopter starting up or jet circling house every 3–4 seconds	

*Interviewed after 9 months of exposure. Family has not moved.
**Away for vacation for 2 weeks during the first 3 months of exposure and 10 days during the month before the interview.

Case Histories 191

Case History J3

Person First son J

Age 13

Pre-exposure health status Good

Health history Normal growth and development

Previous noise exposure No significant

Time to onset of symptoms Immediate for sleep problem; 3–4 months for problems with focus and concentration

	Pre-exposure	During exposure*	Post-exposure**
Sleep	Slept well	Needs "white noise machine" to fall asleep, and more recently MP3 player, too; sleeps well once asleep	Slept well
Headache	No headaches	No change	No change
Cognition	Good, intelligent, gets all A's, finishes home projects	Mother and teachers note distractibility, many grades of B, home projects half done, needs constant reminders for homework and chores; "he just can't seem to focus on anything for more than 5 or 10 minutes"	Organized and persistent about buying presents on vacation
Mood	Good, never "mouthy"	"Snippy, mouthy," talking back, frustrated	Good mood on vacation
Balance/equilibrium	Carsick about once a month	No change	No change
Ear/hearing	Good hearing	No change	No change
Eye/vision	Good with glasses	No change	No change
Other neurological	Normal, no concussion	No change	No change
Cardiovascular	Normal	No change	No change
Gastrointestinal	Normal	No change	No change
Respiratory	Normal, no asthma	No change	No change

*Information provided by parents after 9 months of exposure. Family has not moved.
**Away for vacation for 2 weeks during the first 3 months of exposure and 10 days during the month before the interview.

Case History J4

Person Second son J

Age 8

Pre-exposure health status Good

Health history Normal health and development

Previous noise exposure No significant

Time to onset of symptoms 6 months for mood changes, 7 months for focus problems

	Pre-exposure	During exposure*	Post-exposure**
Sleep	Sleeps very soundly	No change	No change
Headache	No headaches	No change	No change
Cognition	Bright, very focused, gets 100 on every paper	Distracted, getting a few wrong on every paper, teacher noted distraction	Low demand during vacation
Mood	Good, calm, happy	Grumpy, irritable, talking back	Good mood during vacation
Balance/equilibrium	Carsick every 1–2 weeks	No change	Not noted
Ear/hearing	Good hearing	No change	No change
Eye/vision	Good	Just got glasses	No change
Other neurological	Normal, no concussion	No change	No change
Cardiovascular	Normal	No change	No change
Gastrointestinal	Normal	No change	No change
Respiratory	Normal, no asthma	No change	No change

*Information provided by parents after 9 months of exposure. Family has not moved.

**Away for vacation for 2 weeks during the first 3 months of exposure and 10 days during the month before the interview.

FOUR

The REPORT all over again, in plain English for non-clinicians

Abstract and Background

I interviewed 10 families living near large (1.5 to 3 MW) wind turbines, all of which were built since 2004. This gave me 38 people, from infants to age 75. Their symptoms formed a cluster. (See GLOSSARY for clinical terms.)

1) sleep disturbance
2) headache
3) tinnitus (pronounced "tin-uh-tus": ringing or buzzing in the ears)
4) ear pressure
5) dizziness (a general term that includes vertigo, light-headedness, sensation of almost fainting, etc.)
6) vertigo (clinically, vertigo refers to the sensation of spinning, or the room moving)
7) nausea
8) visual blurring
9) tachycardia (rapid heart rate)
10) irritability

11) problems with concentration and memory

12) panic episodes associated with sensations of internal pulsation or quivering, which arise while awake or asleep

People in these families noticed that they developed these symptoms after the turbines started running near their homes. They noticed that when they went away, the symptoms went away. When they came back, the symptoms returned. Eight of the 10 families eventually moved away from their homes because they were so troubled by the symptoms, in some cases abandoning their homes.

Hence the definitive result of my report is that wind turbines cause the symptoms of Wind Turbine Syndrome (WTS). I show this in the common-sense way described above.

Let's clarify something immediately. Not everyone living near turbines gets these symptoms. As a solo, unfunded researcher I could not get the samples needed to figure out what percentages of people at what distances get the symptoms. This needs to be done next. But I could (and did) look at the question of why some people are susceptible and others not, plus who is susceptible, and I used these patterns to explore the *pathophysiology of Wind Turbine Syndrome* (what's going on inside people to cause these specific symptoms).

I would like readers to look at this study—including the detailed accounts I provide of people's experiences around turbines and their health backgrounds—and be able to make their own decisions about whether they should be exposed to these machines.

That said, I was able to prove mathematically that people with pre-existing migraines, motion sensitivity (such as car-sickness or seasickness), or inner-ear damage are especially vulnerable to these symptoms. Equally as interesting, I was able to demonstrate that people with anxiety or other pre-existing mental health problems are not especially susceptible to these symptoms.

 This contradicts wind industry literature, which argues that people who worry about or otherwise dislike the turbines around their homes are the ones getting ill. I show this to be complete nonsense.

Here is what's going on, as I piece together the evidence. *Low frequency noise or vibration tricks the body's balance system into thinking it's moving.* Like seasickness. (It's vital to understand that the human balance system is a complex brain system receiving nerve signals from the inner ears, the eyes, muscles and joints, and inside the chest and abdomen. Because the eyes are involved, visual disturbance from the blades' shadow flicker adds to the balance disturbance.)

Let me repeat this, because its significance is huge. *Low frequency noise or vibration from turbines deceives the body into thinking it's moving.* So what, you say? Not so fast! Research within the last 10 years has demonstrated conclusively that *the way our bodies register balance and motion directly affects an astonishing array of brain functions.*

How? By direct neurologic linkages connecting the organs of balance to various, seemingly unrelated brain functions.

I'll rephrase this, since it's critical to the argument of this report. *The way our bodies perceive balance and motion in turn influences a host of brain functions which at first glance might appear to be entirely unrelated to balance and motion.* As I said, this is what the latest "balance" research tells us—more accurately, balance research combined with psychiatric, neurologic, and cognitive research.

Incidentally, the people specializing in this kind of research are called *otoneurologists* (Europe) and *neurotologists* (United States). (From *oto* for ear, and *neuro* for brain.)

And what are these seemingly unrelated brain functions that are affected by our perception of balance and motion?

1) *Automatic or reflex muscle movements.* These are the well-known vestibulo-ocular reflex, which makes eye movements compensate automatically for head movements, and the vestibulo-collic and vestibulo-spinal reflexes, which dynamically adjust muscle tone in the neck and back to maintain posture during movement.
2) *Alerting.* This consists of attention, alarm, and awakening.
3) *Spatial processing and memory.* Spatial processing is the image-based or pattern-based thinking we use constantly to:
    a) picture things,
    b) remember where things are or where they go,
    c) remember how to get somewhere,
    d) understand how things work,
    e) picture how we want something to turn out,
    f) figure out how to put something together or fix it,

g) figure out the most efficient order and timing of something (such as work around the kitchen, farm, fishing boat, property, or a series of errands),

h) remember what we're looking for when we get someplace (such as errands in town),

i) understand math concepts,

j) and a host of other critical thinking functions.

4) *Physiologic manifestations of fear.* This means fast-pounding heart, increased blood pressure, sweating, nausea, trembling, and hyper-alertness.

5) *Aversive learning.* This is a type of reflex learning whose function is to make creatures avoid potentially harmful things. A classic illustration in both animals and people is vomiting after eating a particular kind of food. We avoid that food for a long time afterwards, even if the food itself was not the cause of the vomiting, and even if it happened only once. (Remember that experience as a child?) This type of learning is so imprinted and automatic that even the environment associated with this experience can trigger the feeling of nausea—like smelling or seeing the particular food, or even approaching the same restaurant. It's an old evolutionary reflex, designed to keep mammals and birds from eating toxic things (with some very interesting consequences for butterfly evolution, but that's another story). What is important here is that we are hardwired to avoid things that make us nauseated.

Okay. *Muscle contractions in eyes and neck and spine, alerting/awakening, spatial processing and memory,* the *physiological manifestations of fear,* and *aversive learning.* All five brain functions are profoundly affected by our sense of balance and motion. All five get messed up when our sense of balance and motion is thrown off.

Back to wind turbines. Open any online newspaper article discussing Wind Turbine Syndrome and you almost invariably discover that someone has posted a comment ridiculing the whole idea for the obvious reason that there's no conceivable way such a disparate range of health problems—memory deficits, spatial processing deficits, anxiety and fear and panic, and aversive learning—could possibly be triggered by a wind turbine, of all things. Preposterous! Clearly, continues our brilliant blogger, people who live near turbines and report these symptoms are making them up (probably because they don't like the darn things), and just as clearly the doctor who takes these complaints seriously (that would be me) is a piker and huckster.

To which I respond: Clearly the authors of these gems of logic are neither neurobiologists nor clinicians—nor are they experiencing the symptoms which are clearly, unambiguously reported by many people living in the shadow (as it were) of industrial wind turbines.

Back to real medicine. The symptoms outlined above occur together *because humans are hardwired to exhibit this precise constellation of symptoms when their balance and motion sensors are disregulated*—as happens to many people living near wind turbines.

It's important to emphasize, these symptoms are not psychological (as if people are fabricating them); they are neurological. People have no control whatsoever over their response to the turbines. It happens automatically. One can't turn on and turn off these symptoms.

We can be emphatic about this because *balance signals* (called *vestibular* signals) *are the one kind of sensory signal we simply cannot tune out*. You can tune out (ignore) what you see and hear, but not what comes in from your sense of balance. Call it a law of nature, if you like.

And what provides our sense of balance? I'm glad you asked. Balance comes from a combination of signals. I'll rephrase this: balance comes from *clusters of signals from different body organs*. One source being, of course, the inner ear.

Stop. We need to review the anatomy of the inner ear. It's essential to understanding Wind Turbine Syndrome.

Start with the weird flap of skin on the side of your head, necessary for holding up your glasses and earrings. This is not the outer ear; it's the pinna. (Boxers get cauliflower pinna.) The outer ear is where you put Q-Tips and where your 2-year-old stores beads and other treasures. It's where earwax lives and where water gets lodged when you shower, and you have to shake it out. The outer ear is a blind pouch ending at the eardrum, sealing off the pouch at the inner end.

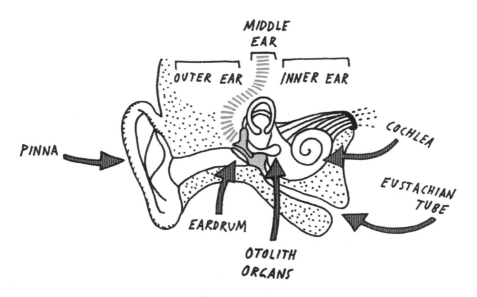

Next comes the middle ear. The place between the eardrum and what's called the oval window. This is the part of the ear that gets infected in little kids. (Moms, remember all those times you took Johnny to the doctor and she said, "Yup, Johnny has an ear infection." This, after Johnny woke up screaming in the night, after having a cold for three days.) The middle ear is open to the air, through the Eustachian tube (pronounced "U-station") from the back of the throat (up behind the nose).

The middle ear houses those three wonderful little bones, incus ("ink-us"), malleus ("mal-ee-us"), and stapes ("stay-peas"), which are linked in a chain. Incus, malleus, and stapes transmit the energy of the vibrating eardrum to the inner ear.

This brings us to our destination. The inner ear (or membranous labyrinth), which consists of the cochlea, the semicircular canals (which you remember from high school biology), and the so-called otolith organs (which you probably don't remember from high school biology).

The otolith organs are key to understanding Wind Turbine Syndrome. They consist of two little membranous sacs, the utricle ("you-trick-ul") and saccule ("sack-ule"), which are attached to the cochlea ("coke-lee-ah," the spiral-shaped, membranous organ that transduces the mechanical energy of sound into neural signals) and to the semicircular canals (membranous organs which make a semi-circle in each of the three planes of movement—vertical forward, vertical sideways, and horizontal—and transduce angular acceleration: when your head is nodding or turning, they detect it).

Embedded in the two otolith organs are—believe it or not—rocks. (*Oto* = ear and *lith* = rock. Remember when your teacher declared you must have rocks in your head?) Well, not really rocks. They're tiny. In fact they're microscopic crystals of calcium carbonate (like calcite or oyster shells), called otoconia ("oto-cone-ia"), stuck together in a mass on top of the patch (macula, pronounced "mack-you-la") of movement-sensing hair cells. The weight and mass of these stones allows the hair cells to detect gravity and linear acceleration.

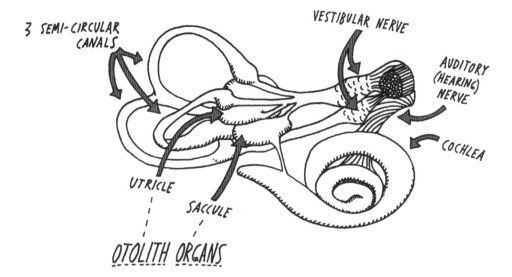

Things now get truly beautiful. Imagine God "with his broad sculptor-hands leaf[ing] through the pages in the dark book of the beginning," showing us the blueprints for the semicircular canals and otolith organs.[1] Structures so fundamental to brain function that they are shared by fish, amphibians, and (so-called) higher vertebrates. Yes, including us. In each of these creatures these organs perform a function not only older than the mind can grasp, but so profound it has come to define what mind itself is. (Note: the cochlea, the organ we use for hearing, evolved much later in mammals.)

We are in the presence of a master key to the mammalian mind. (Not just mammalian, but the entire backboned animal world.) It is this master key, dear reader, that is counterfeited by the low frequency noise from the massive, spinning wind turbine outside your window.

---

[1] Rilke, Rainer Maria. 1991. "The Angels," trans. Snow. *The Book of Images: A Bilingual Edition*, rev. ed. North Point Press, New York, p. 31.

We're in the presence, here, of truly ancient anatomical structures. Many millions of years old. Fish, amphibians, and "higher" vertebrates all have semicircular canals and otolith organs.

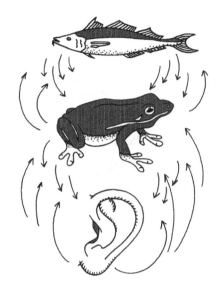

Consider this. Teleost fish, such as cod, hear with their otolith organs. Their otolith organs are their detectors of sound and vibration, such as the movements of nearby predators or prey. Their otolith organs also detect gravity (which way is up) and acceleration (if the fish moves or turns). Atlantic cod otolith organs are so sensitive to water perturbations from infrasound (at 0.1 Hz, or one wave every 10 seconds) that the fish may be able to use seismic sounds from the Mid-Atlantic Ridge or the sounds of waves breaking on distant shores to guide them during migration, hundreds of miles away.

Consider this. In frogs, the saccule (one of the otolith organs) remains the part of the ear most sensitive to substrate-borne vibration. Both the saccule and a newly evolved part of the frog ear, the basilar papilla, detect both sound and vibration, with the saccule capturing lower frequencies and the papilla higher frequencies.

All by way of laying the groundwork for the idea that our own otolith organs have been, ancestrally, detectors of sound, vibration, and low frequency sound, in addition to detecting gravity and body movements. Human otolith organs have retained some of these functions, it turns out: they respond to noise or vibration by sending out vestibular signals.

If stimulated by a loud click or abrupt tone, normal human vestibular organs trigger a measurable, specialized reflex: an electrical signal to muscles in the front of the neck (called the "vestibular evoked myogenic potential" or VEMP). Let me rephrase this, since it's important: a noise, delivered to the ear without any movement of the head or body, sets off a rapid (neural) chain of events that changes neck muscle tone. This neck muscle signal is part of the vestibulo-collic reflex (*collic* meaning "neck," like *collar*). The purpose of the vestibulo-collic reflex is to stabilize the head during body or head movement. *A noise, albeit a loud and distinctive type of noise, sets off a reflex chain of events showing that the vestibular system thinks the body or head is moving, even when it is not. Yes, in normal, healthy adult humans.* (Wind developers, are you reading this?)

Noise doesn't necessarily come in via the air, eardrum, and middle ear, however. Vibrations or "bone-conducted sound" can reach the inner ear directly through the bone in which the inner ear is sculpted. To do this in experiments or as a clinical test, a vibrating object is put against the skin over the mastoid bone behind the ear. It takes less energy (a lower decibel level) to trigger the vestibular response when the signal comes in through bone conduction than when it comes in through the air–middle ear route. Bone conduction also works better at lower sound or vibration frequencies.

Most exciting, *it was shown in 2008 that the normal human vestibular system has a fish- or frog-like sensitivity to low frequency vibration.* In this experiment, a vibrating rod was applied to the skin over the mastoid bone, using carefully calibrated force. Subjects could hear the vibrations as tones, and the researchers detected vestibular responses by measuring electrical signals coming from the subjects' eye muscles. Interesting that this response has a distinct tuning peak at 100 Hz, meaning there is a much bigger vestibular and eye muscle response at 100 Hz than at higher or lower frequencies. (By way of comparison, 100 Hz is equivalent to G-G#, 1½ octaves below middle C. That is, keys 23–24 on a piano.) *At this tuning peak the vibration still produced a measurable vestibular response (eye muscle electrical signals) when the vibration intensity had been reduced so much that the subjects could no longer hear the tones. In fact, the power of the vibration that produced a vestibular response was only about 3% of the power the subjects could hear (15 dB lower).*

This means that some part of the vestibular organs in the inner ear is more sensitive to vibration or bone-conducted sound than the cochlea is. The authors of this study think it's the utricle, one of the two otolith organs, and some special, vibration-sensitive hair cells and nerve fibers that occur mixed in with the other hair cells in the utricle and other vestibular organs.

This is amazing. (It would be heretical if it hadn't been shown in a well-conducted experiment.) It has been gospel among acousticians for the past 70 years that if a person can't hear a sound, it's too weak for it to be detected or registered by any other part of the body. We can now write this as follows: ~~If a person can't hear a sound, it's too weak for it to be detected or registered by any other part of the body.~~ Because it turns out it's wrong. (It also means that using the A-weighted network for community noise studies is probably outdated. See p. 214.)

> And silent be,
> That through the channels of the ear
> May wander like a river
> The swaying sound of the sea.
>
> —W. H. Auden, from "Look, Stranger"

Back, now, to what provides us with our sense of balance. I said balance comes from a combination of signals, and I just explained how some of them originate in the inner ear. Besides the inner ear, the eyes also send motion and position signals to the brain. So, too, do muscles and joints all over the body, involving what are called "stretch" receptors, telling us where we are in space.

And lastly, we maintain our balance by newly discovered stretch and pressure receptors in the chest and abdomen. These tiny receptors use various organs, including blood vessels and the blood in them, as weights or masses to detect the body's orientation to gravity and other forms of acceleration.

The foregoing is the proper context for studying people's health complaints from wind turbines. Health complaints that are routinely dismissed by the wind industry as nonsense. (Not unlike the tobacco industry dismissing health issues from smoking.) The wind industry, however, is not composed of clinicians, nor is it made up of people suffering from wind turbines.

My hope is that researchers will soon be able to measure and correlate wind turbine audible and sub-audible noise, and vibration, with the symptoms people experience in real time—that is, while they're actually experiencing the symptoms. (This has been done for similar complaints in published cases, as described below.) Until that happens, I offer this report as a pilot study.

Introduction and More Background

Developers say turbines are quiet. No louder than a household refrigerator. With this patently false claim, they easily convince local governments it's okay to erect turbines mere hundreds of feet from people's homes. Nearly in their backyards, in many instances.

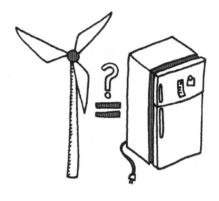

Wind turbine setbacks, in other words, are wind industry–driven. There is virtually no government regulation.

This is where my phone (and email) starts ringing. People from around the world contacting me to say, often with great emotion in their voice, that they haven't slept well (if at all) since the turbines were installed 1500 feet (and more) from their back door. Not just insomnia, but a host of health issues, again, since the turbines in the neighbor's field began operation.

For over four years I've been listening to these complaints. People describing symptoms that are remarkably consistent, person to person. Consistent and, often, debilitating. Symptoms, I began realizing, that suggest people's balance systems are getting scrambled.

I realized what's needed is a clinical definition of the way people are getting sick when they live near wind turbines. If the symptoms form a coherent cluster that makes physiologic sense, we're in a better position to figure out:

a) precisely what's causing it
b) how many people are getting it
c) who is susceptible
d) how to control or prevent it

This became my goal: figure out the pathophysiology of the illness cluster they all describe.

Except immediately there's a problem. Which is that developers focus on noise. They hire an acoustician to measure noise levels (incidentally, there are many ways to slice and dice noise measurements), who then writes a report saying, in effect,

a) the turbines are emitting this (whatever) dB of noise
b) the conventional acoustical wisdom about this range of dB says it doesn't create health problems
c) hence, we conclude these people are faking their symptoms
d) end of story

I turn the above sequence on its head. We need to begin with c) *symptoms*, not a) *noise levels*. The symptoms are consistent person to person, whether it's England or Canada or what have you. Furthermore, the symptom cluster fits with known clinical mechanisms. There is no mystery here.

Hence, the symptom cluster becomes—must become—the chief reference point.

When measuring noise, one must refine one's measurements so as to answer what the precise qualities of the noise spectrum are, *at this moment, when people are actually getting symptoms*, versus that other moment when they're not getting symptoms. *This* is the value of noise measurements.

Other published reports on health and wind turbines, by the way, find the identical set of symptoms to what I found. In my report I review papers by Dr. Amanda Harry, Barbara Frey and Peter Hadden, and Prof. Robyn Phipps.

1) Harry found all the same problems. By limiting her sample to people who were having symptoms, she came up with a group shifted toward older folks. This suggests that older age is a risk factor.

2) Frey and Hadden document the same symptoms in people's own narratives.

3) Phipps mailed questionnaires to everyone living within 9.3 miles of turbines. All her respondents lived at least 1.24 miles (2 km) away from turbines. She got positive responses about unpleasant physical symptoms from 2%. She got spontaneous phone calls from nearly 7%, who wanted to tell her more specifically about their distress and problems from turbine noise and vibration—most of them with disturbed sleep. Yes, even at these distances—more than 2 km or 1¼ miles.

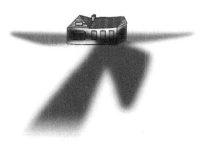

My own subjects make it clear their problems are caused by noise and vibration and, in some instances, moving blade shadows. What's more, my subjects notice that their symptoms come and go according to the wind's direction and strength, blade spinning speed, which way the turbines are facing, and particular sounds coming from the turbines. In other words, they see their symptoms increase and decrease depending on what the turbines are doing. They also know that the quality of noise is strange and bothersome even compared to other types of noise, like nearby trains or traffic. A few people were specifically bothered by shadow flicker in rooms or blade shadows sweeping the landscape.

Above all, the symptoms went away when my subjects left home and the turbines, and returned when they came back home. Ultimately, most of the study subjects left their homes for good.

Again, the only rational way to study the problem is *symptoms first, noise measurements second*, not the reverse.

Noise. You, dear reader, need to understand what noise is before we go further. If you're confident your grasp of noise is sophisticated, then skip the next few paragraphs. Otherwise, here we go.

Wind turbines make noise from infrasonic (below what we can hear), through the range we can hear (audible, in other words), to ultrasonic (above what we can hear). This is well established. By "above" and "below" we mean "pitch." "Frequency" means "pitch." Hence, low frequency noise (LFN) means "low-pitched," like the low notes on a piano. High frequency means high-pitched, like the "s" sounds in human speech. Frequency is expressed in Hertz (Hz), which means "waves or cycles per second."

Noise also has a property of intensity or power which, if the sound is within the hearing range, we call "loudness." Loudness or intensity is measured as "decibels" or "sound pressure level." These are both measures of how much energy, or power, is in the sound wave, and is also called "amplitude."

Next definition: wavelength. A high frequency wave means a short wavelength (think of ocean waves: when the waves arrive in rapid succession, the distance between the wave peaks is short). Low frequency means a long wavelength: the peaks are farther apart, though the waves travel at the same speed in the same medium.

Now things get interesting. *A sound wave in the air is a sequence of pressure changes.* A sound wave in a solid is more like a vibration. (In fact the word "vibration" is technically used to refer only to what happens in solids.)

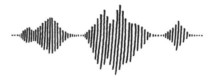

As an aside, I will often talk about noise and vibration together because I'm talking about a continuum of energy as it passes through different substances. For example a sound wave coming through the air, hitting a building, can make the walls vibrate, which in turn sets up sound waves inside the room. Or vibrations coming through the earth may set up vibrations in a building, which may in turn set up sound waves in a room or may be transmitted to the ear by bone conduction. (For low frequencies, there are a lot of these sorts of energy exchanges. The energy doesn't get attenuated or diminished so much with distance or passing through things, but tends to keep going.)

When symptoms of the sort we're dealing with have been medically studied, they are typically associated with lower sound frequency ranges—below hearing range or in the lower part of the hearing range. (I review two studies of this sort on pp. 106–8 in the REPORT FOR CLINICIANS.) With further research into Wind Turbine Syndrome, it may turn out that some of the turbine noise in the higher frequencies is also creating symptoms; however, the chief noise culprit, from studies of similar symptoms, appears to be low frequency noise.

Loudness, or intensity, also matters. Acousticians with the wind industry argue that because the intensity of low frequency noise from turbines is below the usual air-borne human hearing thresholds, then it's too weak to have health effects. Acousticians are taught, "*If you can't hear it, it can't hurt you!*" This, however, is an oversimplification of how the body works (as described above, in the section on how sound triggers vestibular reflexes). Noise health standards focus on protecting people's ears from loud noise that could damage hearing, yet ignore other harmful effects of lower sound levels (as documented, for example, in the extensive literature on night noise, stress hormones, and cardiovascular changes).

When we decide to look at symptoms first, the noise issue in Wind Turbine Syndrome becomes simple. People's symptoms come and go. Acousticians need to measure noise levels when symptoms are present and compare these to noise levels when symptoms are absent. In this manner they can find out exactly *what frequencies* at *what intensities* are causing symptoms.

In the Discussion section of my REPORT FOR CLINICIANS I give two examples of published accounts by German noise control engineers, correlating symptoms with their noise measurements. In each case the symptoms (very similar to Wind Turbine Syndrome, incidentally) were due to very low frequency noise. In one case the noise was identified but not the noise source; in the other the source was a large building ventilator fan.

Back to my crash course on noise. (Yes, pun intended.) Resonance. Resonance is what happens inside the body of a guitar or violin after a string is plucked or disturbed by a bow. It's like an echo inside a space. Thus, certain wavelengths bounce back and forth very efficiently, given the size of that space. The walls of the space tend to vibrate at particular frequencies, and if the natural vibration frequency of the wall is the same as the frequency of the bouncing sound, the wall itself (guitar wall, violin wall) can give an added "punch" to the sound waves at its "resonant frequency," making these frequencies louder.

This is a lot like pumping a swing. (We all did this as children.) Swinging is a kind of wave function, like sound, with frequency and amplitude. The frequency of the swing is how many times per minute it's going back and forth. Frequency depends on the length of the ropes—a short swing swings faster. Amplitude is how high the child is swinging. Resonance is a child who knows how to pump (add some energy to the swinging) at exactly the right time to increase the amplitude (swing higher). The frequency stays the same, but, as the child pumps, she swings higher and higher.

The child pumping is like the wall of a resonant chamber; it provides a little push to the "wave" at exactly the right time.

Okay, course on noise is over. Now let's apply it to Wind Turbine Syndrome.

Resonances occur inside body spaces and in solid but flexible or elastic parts of the body, such as along the spine. Different parts of the body have different resonant frequencies. Many of these are in the low frequency range. When a sound wave or vibration hits the body, it's more likely to set up vibrations in a body part with a matching resonant frequency.

In Wind Turbine Syndrome, an important body resonance is the resonance of the chest and abdominal space. The chest wall is made of elastic muscles, bones, cartilage, tendons, and ligaments, giving the chest a natural recoil we use in breathing. We use energy to expand the chest to breathe in, but much of the force needed to push the air back out occurs effortlessly from the elastic recoil of the chest.

One of the important parts of the breathing mechanism is the diaphragm muscle at the bottom of the chest. It's dome-shaped, like the top of an egg. When you take a breath, the diaphragm flattens. As it flattens, it pulls down, thus expanding the chest space and pushing on the abdominal space. The abdominal space is very soft and flexible, the front being thin sheets of muscle, skin, and other soft tissues, without bone or cartilage. So when you breathe in, your stomach sticks out. When you relax the diaphragm muscle, it springs back to its dome shape and it pushes air out. Natural elasticity at work.

Hence, when air pressure waves enter the lung, it takes very little energy in the air pressure waves to set this very mobile system vibrating. At frequencies between 4 and 8 times per second (or Hz, which means "times per second"), the diaphragm will vibrate. Frequencies of 4–8 Hz are low frequency noise or infrasound, below hearing range.

Not only does the diaphragm vibrate, but the entire mass of internal organs in the abdomen swings up and down, towards and away from the lungs. One of the largest abdominal organs, the liver, is attached to the underside of the diaphragm.

There are other places in the body with resonance, including the eyes (globes with bone around them and less dense material inside) and the brain case. The inner-ear researchers who discovered the 100 Hz peak for vestibular response talk about the skull resonance at 500 Hz, where the skull "rings." Even the spine (backbone) has a resonance frequency. The spine is elastic. If it's vibrated at a particular frequency it can set up a vertical vibration along the spine.

Even very small body parts, like the organs of the inner ear, have resonances or peak responses that depend on their size, stiffness, and the pressure of the fluid on either side. Like that 100 Hz peak response of the utricle.

In sum, what we casually call *noise* can have a powerful impact on numerous internal structures and cavities. We will see the significance of all this in the Discussion, below.

Before moving on to the Methods section, a few words about measuring sound power and what's called "A-weighting" and "C-weighting." It's difficult to measure the loudness 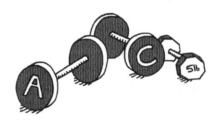 (energy) of sound in consistent, reproducible ways, especially at low frequencies. A-weighted and C-weighted "networks," in sound-measuring equipment, screen energy (loudness) according to frequency. To come up with a single number for the loudness of noise, the contributions of many frequencies must be added together. The weighting network controls how much each frequency contributes to the number.

The A-weighting network is the usual one for studies of community noise, perhaps more out of tradition than good sense. It's designed to duplicate the frequency response of human hearing—human hearing via air, the outer ear, tympanic membrane, and three bones of the middle ear. This outer-to-middle ear (A-weighted) system is a filter that emphasizes the high sounds used in human speech recognition, while de-emphasizing, or indeed only minimally capturing, the contributions of mid- and lower-range audible sounds, as well as infrasound (defined as 20 Hz and below). A-weighting slightly enhances the contributions of sounds in the 1000 to 6000 Hz range (on the piano: from C two octaves *above* middle C, key 64, to F# *above the highest note* on the piano), and progressively reduces the contributions of lower frequencies below about 800 Hz (G-G# 1½ octaves *above* middle C, keys 59–60, hardly a low note). At 100 Hz, where the human vestibular organ has a highly sensitive response to vibration (G-G# 1½ octaves below middle C, keys 23–24), an A-weighted measurement captures only 1/1000 of the sound energy actually present (−30 dB). At 31 Hz (B, the second-to-bottom white key, key 3), A-weighting captures only 1/10,000 of the sound energy present (−40 dB). At 10 Hz, a frequency found in another study to cause Wind Turbine Syndrome–like symptoms (see p. 106 in REPORT FOR CLINICIANS), A-weighting captures only 10^{-7}, or one ten-millionth, of the sound energy present.

The C-weighting network, on the other hand, has a flat response over the audible range—meaning, it does not enhance or reduce the contributions of the different audible sound frequencies—and a well-defined decreasing response below 31 Hz. At 10 Hz, C-weighting captures 1/25 of the sound energy present. Like A-weighting, it is standard on sound measuring equipment.

C-weighting makes far more sense for describing community noise than A-weighting, because A-weighting is biased towards high-pitched sounds—the very sounds that walls filter out, hence the ones least likely to bother a person on the other side of a wall from a noise source. The sounds that get through walls are the low ones—the rumbly undertones of a TV or people talking in the next room, the thump of footsteps or a washer running overhead, the rumble of a snowplow outside, or the kid's boom car a block away. These sounds may even create new vibrations in walls or windows. It's odd that by using A-weighting, community noise measurements (including wind turbine noise measurements) concentrate on the very frequencies that a little insulation easily gets rid of.

Now that we know that inaudible, bone-conducted tones at 100 Hz still stimulate the human vestibular system (as described above), there is little justification for using A-weighting in studies of community noise—by itself, that is. Used together with C-weighting, the difference between A and C measurements of the same noise provides a consistent and easily available way to estimate the power of lower frequency sounds in the noise.

It's easy to obtain standardized measuring equipment with either A- or C-weighting networks, but measuring the power of the lowest frequency sounds requires expensive and specialized equipment that's not standardized among models. Nevertheless, if we are to fully understand Wind Turbine Syndrome, it's at this lowest of low frequencies that measurements must be made.

Methods

I used what's called a *case series* as my research protocol. (Remember my definition of a case series from WHY I WROTE THIS: "*A descriptive account of a series of individuals with the same new medical problem.*")

In medical research, *case series* don't usually have control (comparison) groups. However, I added a new wrinkle to my study, based on my training in field ecology: despite not having a formal control (comparison) group, I chose subjects and arranged the way I collected information so I could create comparisons.

First, to call this a wind-turbine-associated problem at all, I compared how people were *during exposure* to how they were when *not exposed*, and
I specified that "not exposed" meant both *before* and *after* living near turbines. *All my subjects saw their problems start soon after*

turbines went on-line near their homes, and all saw their problems go away when they were away from the turbines.

Second, I compared subjects who exhibited particular symptoms to those who did not. Then I looked at whether these differences were influenced by age, underlying health conditions, etc., to discover medical risk factors.

There was a third type of implicit comparison going on—to the population at large. For example, Dr. Harry and I sampled in a similar way—by interviewing affected adults—and we both wound up with samples shifted toward people in their 50's or older. This suggests that older people are more often affected, since older people are over-represented in our samples. (This makes medical sense, and also corresponds to who is most bothered by noise in other, non-wind-turbine settings.)

Additionally, in my study there are more people with underlying migraine than in the general population, suggesting that people with migraine are, like older people, more susceptible.

Now let's consider how epidemiologic studies of Wind Turbine Syndrome might look and what they might show, as distinct from my *case series* approach. There are several types of epidemiologic study.

In a prospective or longitudinal study, a scientist begins by defining two identical groups to be studied, *before* either group is exposed to a (supposedly) disease-causing or disease-improving agent. One group is called the *study group*, and the other the *control group*. The study group is the individuals about to be exposed to the agent. The control group is identical in every conceivable way to the study group: by age, sex, income, education, etc.

Then exposure starts. The researchers monitor what happens to everybody in both groups, make comparisons, do statistics, and draw conclusions.

Prospective studies are used when exposure is likely to make a person better, as in clinical trials for new medications. The progress of the subjects in each group is monitored carefully and data analyzed along the way, to make sure the supposedly helpful agent is not actually harmful (this sometimes happens, and then clinical trials are stopped midway through).

Prospective studies can also be used when people expose themselves to the harmful agent, as in smoking, or when something happens that has been arranged for other reasons, like closing an airport in one location and opening a new one in another location (this was a real study, showing the detrimental effects of noise exposure on children's reading). But it would be, of course, unethical to design a study to expose people to something already suspected to be harmful.

A cross-sectional study is different from a prospective or longitudinal study. A cross-sectional study compares exposed (*study*) to non-exposed (*control*) people during the same time period—individuals living or working in different places, depending on where the exposure occurs. Choosing the study populations is difficult, since the two groups need to be the same in every way except the exposure. Another difficult part is deciding what to measure and how to measure it. For example, with wind turbines, the type of in-depth clinical interviews I used would not be feasible for sample sizes of hundreds or thousands of people. On the other hand, mail-out surveys, while potentially reaching entire populations, have the problems of poor response rates and potential misunderstanding of the questions, both of which introduce bias. Survey questions are often pretty bland and simplified to make sure everyone understands them the same way, and to avoid being suggestive.

At the end of the REPORT FOR CLINICIANS I talk about what kind of studies might be feasible or desirable as a next step, especially designs that combine specific, realistic health data with broad population coverage. Select European countries may be ideal for this approach—those that have both wind turbines and unified health systems in which the diagnosis for every visit to every physician is recorded in the same central database.

Back to my report. The problem in any clinical study is figuring out which new symptoms are due to a new exposure and which are not. In an epidemiologic study this is worked out by having parallel groups, with one group not exposed. Since I didn't have the resources to do such a study, I insisted that among my study subjects there be a post-exposure period—a time after exposure ended, during which the symptoms disappeared. *Wind Turbine Syndrome is defined only as those symptoms which came on during exposure and abated only after exposure ended.* It may not capture all the health effects of wind turbine exposure, because of the limitations built into my study design. But it certainly captured a significant set of symptoms.

There's an additional way I generated comparison groups. I collected information on all family members during the interviews—about themselves, their children, and disabled family members who could not be interviewed. In this way I discovered that not everyone in each family was equally affected, despite living in the same house at the same distance from the turbines. I used comparisons among affected and non-affected people to figure out which parts of their pre-exposure medical histories predicted which symptoms during exposure.

With this in mind, notice how I chose my study subjects:

1) at least one family member was severely affected by living near turbines
2) the family either had to have left the home or spent sufficient time away to experience relief from symptoms
3) the people I interviewed had to be able to say clearly, consistently, and in detail what had happened to them, under what conditions and at what time
4) they all lived near turbines put into operation between 2004 and 2007
5) if they had already moved out when interviewed, it was less than 6 weeks since they'd moved out
6) they had to have taken serious action to protect themselves from the turbine exposure (generally identified as noise):
   a) some moved out
   b) some purchased a second home in anticipation of moving out
   c) some left home for months
   d) one family renovated the house in an effort to mitigate the noise
   e) one man took to sleeping in his root cellar

A final point. This squiggly symbol, χ^2, is called "chi squared" (pronounced "keye," as in "eye"). Don't panic! It's a simple statistical test. I'll illustrate with an example.

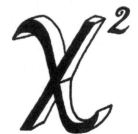

1) You have a group of people.
2) You classify each one as tall or short, with blue eyes or brown eyes.

3) A χ^2 statistic lets you say if blue eyes are associated with being tall or short in anything other than a random (unrelated) way.

4) Since everyone knows that having blue or brown eyes has nothing to do with being tall or short, if you do a χ^2 statistic on, say, 20 people, each categorized for both of these qualities (eye color and height), it would come out to be non-significant.

5) End of illustration.

Now, that wasn't so hard, was it?

Notice when you read my clinical report that you will encounter what are called p (probability) values in parentheses, together with χ^2 values. Again, don't panic. The p is the probability that the relationship between the two variables (eye color and height) is random. In other words, that being tall does not increase your probability of having eyes of one color or the other, or that height and eye color are totally unrelated.

Values of p vary between low numbers close to 0 and 1. Low p values mean *there's a significant correlation between the two variables.* "Low" would be less than 0.05. "Very low," or less than 0.01, means there's an even stronger likelihood the two variables (e.g., eye color and height) occur together more than by chance.

Okay, you can breathe again; we're done with the math. This is precisely how I identify "risk factors" in my study. (Risk factor is something in your medical history or makeup that makes you susceptible, in this case, to Wind Turbine Syndrome when exposed to turbines.) I apply a χ^2 analysis. For instance, I look at whether a person has or does not have tinnitus when exposed to turbines. I compare that to whether the person does or doesn't have a history of industrial noise exposure. I discovered, in this particular example, that a significant relationship does exist.

We'll come back to this in the Results section, below.

Results

My study demonstrated the following to be the core symptoms of Wind Turbine Syndrome.

1) First, *almost everyone had disturbed sleep*. Two particularly interesting patterns emerged in the disturbed sleep.

    a) The first was a "fear" pattern of arousal or awakening, including childhood night terrors and adults waking up alarmed and hyper-alert. These adults felt they had to check to see if someone had broken into the home, even though they knew they had been awakened by turbine noise. Some adults woke up with a racing heart at night or feeling not able to breathe.

    b) The second was a tendency to urinate a lot at night. For adults this meant getting up frequently, and for one child it involved bed wetting (which resolved whenever she was away from the turbines).

    I didn't look for risk factors for sleep disturbance since virtually everyone interviewed had disturbed sleep.

2) *Headaches.* Slightly more than half the study subjects had headaches that were worse than what that person normally experienced before and after turbine exposure (what we call "at baseline"). The headaches were more frequent, more severe, and lasted longer than that individual's usual headaches (the person's baseline headaches).

Half of the subjects who had worsened headaches were people with pre-existing migraine disorder (i.e., a hereditary tendency to get severe headaches along with dizziness, nausea, visual changes, or avoidance of light, noise, or movement during headaches). All the children in the study who got headaches during turbine exposure either had migraine disorder themselves or were the children of parents with migraine disorder.

About half the adults who got headaches during exposure had no risk factors for headache that I could identify. This suggests that anyone can get severe headaches when exposed to turbines.

3) *Ear symptoms.* Tinnitus was a dominant symptom during exposure. Tinnitus: ringing, a tone, buzzing, or a waterfall noise from one or both ears, or even a buzzing that seems to be inside the head. Risk factors for tinnitus during exposure were:

   a) having some tinnitus before exposure (the tinnitus during exposure was worse)
   b) having some hearing loss before exposure
   c) a previous industrial noise exposure

All these suggest previous damage to the inner ear, which could come from noise exposure, chemotherapy, certain antibiotics, or other causes.

People also experienced pain and popping and a feeling of pressure in their ears, and some shifts in hearing.

4) The fourth core symptom I am calling VVVD, for *Visceral Vibratory Vestibular Disturbance*. This is a new symptom to medicine, I believe. Before reading further, you should read the VVVD symptom accounts in the REPORT FOR CLINICIANS (pp. 55–59), so you have a mental picture of what people say they experience. Once you've looked over those accounts we can move on to consider how the symptoms of VVVD can occur together, the symptoms being:

   a) A feeling of internal pulsation, quivering or vibration. For some, breathing feels controlled or restricted.

   b) Nervousness or jitteriness. Fear. The urge to flee. The urge to check the house for safety.

   c) Shaking

   d) Rapid heartbeat

   e) Nausea

VVVD is essentially the *symptoms of a panic attack associated with feelings of movement inside the chest in people who have never had panic attacks before* (none of my subjects had).

Because VVVD is so similar to panic attacks, I looked for a correlation between VVVD and a history of any other kind of anxiety or depression or mental health disorder. I found no such relationship. However *there was a highly significant correlation between VVVD and pre-existing motion sensitivity* (i.e., people who get car-sick, seasick, or had a history of repeated episodes of vertigo).

Out of the 21 adults (age 22 and up) in the study, 14 had VVVD. The two toddlers in the study looked like they had something similar. Though we don't know exactly what they felt, they woke up screaming several times per night, and were inconsolable and hard to get back to bed or to sleep. The two 5-year-olds in the study also awoke fearful in the night.

5) *Concentration and memory.* Almost everyone in the study had some kind of problem with concentration and memory. The more severe concentration problems were linked with a general loss of energy and motivation. What's noteworthy among many of my subjects is the degree to which they lost basic skills they had prior to turbine exposure, and the way teachers noticed new problems with kids' schoolwork and sent notes home. (Be sure you read the Concentration and Memory symptom accounts in the REPORT FOR CLINICIANS, pp. 61–64, and the accounts of recovery from these symptoms, pp. 65–66).

For some people, these problems with thinking resolved as soon as they got away from the turbines, or even if the turbines turned in another direction. For others, they did not resolve immediately but improved gradually over time. Sleep deprivation undoubtedly plays a large role in the memory and concentration difficulties, but these patterns of recovery suggest an additional influence, which may be the direct influence of vestibular disturbance on various forms of thinking (see the Discussion, below).

6) The remaining core symptoms were *irritability and anger*, which occurred in most of my subjects, including the children. Often it was the children's behavior and school problems, their irritability and loss of social coping skills, that drove families to move out of their homes and away from the turbines.

7) Most subjects had *fatigue*—sometimes a distinctly leaden feeling—*and loss of enjoyment and motivation for usual activities*. For most this cleared up soon after they got away from the turbines.

8) Finally, I listed clusters of symptoms that subjects told me about, but which would require other modes of study (including physical exams and testing, and a case-control format) to find out if they are connected to turbines. These symptoms occurred in low numbers in my study. They included *lower respiratory infections* (bronchitis, pneumonia, pleurisy) that were unusual for the people who got them, *worsened asthma, unusual middle ear fluid or infections,* and *ocular stroke.*

Though my study cannot prove a connection, I think they are worth attention in a large-scale study of wind turbine health effects.

Discussion

This section is about how I think Wind Turbine Syndrome works, and the ideas I got from the medical literature and my referees. This is the most interesting section—where we join the dots.

I originally recognized the symptoms of Wind Turbine Syndrome as being something coherent—something that hangs together—because I already knew about what's called *migrainous vertigo* or *migraine-anxiety associated dizziness*.

Migraine is not just a bad headache. It is a neurologic syndrome with many other peculiar symptoms associated with it. My husband has had migraines since he was a teen, but he never gets headaches. He gets dizziness, tiredness, and patches where he can't see (scotoma). He has to lie down till it goes away. Some years ago he had a terrible episode of nauseating vertigo (a spinning kind of dizziness), tinnitus, and anxiety that developed into depression. The person who figured out what was wrong with him was the otolaryngologist to whom this book is dedicated, Dr. Dudley Weider.

Dr. Weider taught me how migraine, vertigo, tinnitus, and anxiety are neurologically related—and he treated my husband successfully. I might add that my husband has always been motion sensitive. This is true for about half of the people with migraine.

Thus, when I started hearing about the symptoms in Wind Turbine Syndrome, I recognized it as a related complex of symptoms. I had hoped to share this report with Dr. Weider, but, alas, he had passed away. Instead I had the pleasure of sharing it with a group of his former colleagues in otolaryngology. (Read through the list of referees and readers of this report. It's a Dudley Weider festschrift.) They taught me many other important matters regarding balance and the inner ear, which I've incorporated into this report.

Drs. Lehrer and Black recognized the symptom complex of Wind Turbine Syndrome as similar to the symptoms of an inner-ear problem called endolymphatic hydrops (EH). In the case of EH the symptoms are continuous or vary for unknown reasons. In Wind Turbine Syndrome these symptoms come and go depending on whether people are near or far from the turbines, or whether the turbines are making a particular kind of noise or facing in certain directions.

EH, which includes Meniere's Disease (pronounced "Muh-nears") and perilymphatic fistula (where fluid is leaking from the inner ear into the middle ear), involves distorted pressure relationships between the two fluid compartments in the inner ear: the endolymph (inside the membranous labyrinth) and perilymph (around the membranous labyrinth, between it and the bony canals). This causes erratic and distorted balance and, often, distorted hearing signals to be sent to the brain.

Beyond the dizziness and hearing problems, EH is commonly known (among doctors who assess this problem) to be associated with difficulties with short-term memory, concentration, multitasking, arithmetic, and reading. There can also be headache, sleep disturbance, and marked mental performance deficiencies compared to baseline.

Sounds like Wind Turbine Syndrome without the turbines.

Interestingly, low frequency noise exposure (for a short time, at high but non-traumatizing intensities in guinea pigs) causes temporary EH. (What about continuous amounts of low frequency noise at lower intensities in humans, one wonders?) The experimental low frequency noise exposure also made the animals temporarily more sensitive to noise, called "hyperacusis," another effect seen in the Wind Turbine Syndrome study. And EH is experienced in people as a sense of fullness or pressure in the ears, a common symptom in the current study.

This brings us to the balance system and how it works. The balance system is a complex system that penetrates many areas of the brain and draws sensory signals from all over the body. Other senses have only one kind of sensory input; the balance system has four.

By balance system I mean both a) *how the body maintains its upright posture* and b) *everything to do with motion and position awareness*. For example, the balance system is highly active during the turns and twists of diving or gymnastics, even though a person is not staying upright.

Why all this focus on the balance system? Because I think that *people susceptible to imbalance are especially susceptible to Wind Turbine Syndrome*. So I need to explain the different ways people become unbalanced, so to be able to explain how the air pressure variations (sound) or vibrations from wind turbines may be triggering an abnormal sense of motion or instability in susceptible people.

As I mentioned before, *motion* and *position* signals come from four discrete body systems and are integrated by balance centers (vestibular centers) in the brain:

1) eyes (visual system)
2) motion- and position-sensing organs in the inner ear (vestibular system)
3) stretch receptors from muscles and joints all over the body, and touch receptors in the skin (somato-sensory system)
4) stretch and pressure receptors associated with organs in the chest and abdomen

The balance system requires that at least two of the first three channels (visual, vestibular, and somato-sensory) be working and providing harmonious data at every moment if we are to maintain balance. Hang onto this point; it's extremely important. We might call it the *Law of Balance*.

For example, the vestibular organs in the inner ear tend not to work so well in older folks. If the inner ear is not sending correct signals, people are more dependent on what they can see and on what their feet and legs are feeling to keep their balance.

Since two channels have to be sending harmonious signals for balance to work, these people are in trouble in the dark.

If you have good balance, try this experiment: stand on one foot and feel all the little corrective movements your foot and ankle are making to keep you upright. People with normal balance can stand on one foot indefinitely.

Now close your eyes. See how long before you have to put your other foot down to keep from falling over.

You can't keep your balance in this situation because you've deprived yourself of both vision and adequate somato-sensory input from the legs—and one system, the vestibular input from the inner ear, is not enough. (If you don't have good balance, keep both feet on the floor when you close your eyes, and you may still notice a difference.)

How this clinical rule will incorporate the new fourth channel of balance information—visceral gravity and motion detection—remains to be seen. It may be that brain vestibular centers also take account of the amounts and quality of information coming from each channel, not just whether a channel is active. For example, when visual information is lacking (eyes closed, or in the dark), the extra somato-sensory information from even a finger against a wall or railing can be enough to make a person feel stable and comfortable. Likewise it's easier to keep your balance on two feet than on one. Balance is harder on two feet if the feet are lined up end to end on a balance beam or, worse, on a moving and unstable tightrope. All these situations limit or degrade the somato-sensory information coming from the legs and feet, but do not reduce it to zero.

Variations in balance function seem to fall into four broad categories:

1) *The first is very young age.* Little children fall down a lot. As kids get older and improve their balance, they can do more

complex things without falling. At very young ages children are mapping their entire sensory system onto the world. For example, an infant figures out how far he has to reach his arm to touch something, and what that looks and feels like. This gives him a sense of distance, mapping that concept of distance onto his visual sensors and the coordinated stretch receptors of his arm and shoulder.

This process of learning where the parts of the body are in space, through increasingly complex activities, continues through childhood. In its early stages, children are more susceptible to balance disturbance.

2) *A second origin of balance variation is differences in the central (brain) processing of balance and motion-related signals.* People who are motion sensitive, which includes about half of people with migraine disorder, as well as other people, have difficulty successfully integrating the signals from the different sensory channels of balance. Their brains tend to over-emphasize or under-emphasize certain channels.

For example, in a person with migrainous vertigo and tinnitus—like my husband—the signals from the inner ear may be turned up too loud. So, centrally, the brain has to turn these down. It has to deal with the over-intensity of one signal. Or it may not be that they're too loud, but distorted, in which case the brain needs to down-weight the signals from that channel even more.

When we turn down the signals from the inner ear, we become more dependent on the visual channel or the somato-sensory channel. People who are visually dependent for balance are often afraid of heights (witness my husband).

This is because, when everything is far away, there's less visual position information that can be drawn from what one sees (less retinal slip and parallax changes as one moves, for example). Fear is associated with this experience because instability or uncertainty about position in space leads to fear in a reflex neurologic way (more on this later).

Someone who is surface dependent, on the other hand, may be in more trouble when the surface is slippery, because he relies more on the position information coming from his muscles and joints. These signals are distorted by the slippery surface.

3) *The third source of balance variation or dysfunction is inner-ear damage, or congenital or developmental malformations of the inner ear.* Damage may come from loud noise or blast exposures, head or neck injury (including "minor" ones like concussion or whiplash), complications of repeated or chronic middle ear infections in childhood, or exposure to certain chemicals (aminoglycoside antibiotics or chemotherapy with cisplatin, for example). There is also endolymphatic hydrops (EH), the inner-ear pathology (described above) that includes Meniere's disease and perilymphatic fistula. Autoimmune disorders like lupus (in which the body's own antibodies attack parts of the body) can also cause endolymphatic hydrops, as can natural variations in how the bones and channels of the inner ear are formed, or such differences combined with trauma or other forms of injury.

4) *The fourth source of balance variation or dysfunction is older age.* There seems to be deterioration of inner-ear function after about age 50, varying among people, of course.

This brings us to *compensated* vs. *uncompensated balance dysfunction*. If you happen to have a balance dysfunction and yet are able to compensate for it, you feel fine. You keep your balance. Your body is confident of where it is in space. On the other hand if there's an additional challenge, or distortion from a second channel, then you're off balance—you feel unsteady or dizzy, or have vertigo or motion sickness. This is *uncompensated balance dysfunction*. The vestibular or balance centers in the brain, which have the job of integrating all the different signals of the balance system, can ignore or suppress signals from one channel that don't match the others, *but they can't for two channels*. One functioning channel is not enough.

People who suffer from Wind Turbine Syndrome have, I believe, a compensated balance problem at baseline (meaning before exposure, in their usual state of health), in one of the four ways described above. *Exposure to wind turbines pushes them over the edge, since the brain can't ignore disorienting signals from two channels at once.* At least one set of false signals is now coming from the turbines. The other problem is in any of the four categories described immediately above.

But how can false balance signals come from wind turbines? *By disturbing any of the four sensory channels for balance, hijacking that channel into sending discordant signals that the vestibular centers in the brain can't integrate. Or by disturbing several channels at once.*

The four ways of disturbing the four balance channels are:

1) Inner-ear (vestibular organ) disturbance: Low frequency noise or vibration stimulates the otolith organs, stimulating vestibular (balance) brain centers (as described in the first section of this chapter), and producing illusory self-

movement, unsteadiness, neck muscle tightening via the vestibulo-collic reflex, and other symptoms. When ear symptoms (such as pressure, popping, tinnitus, pain, or hearing changes) are prominent, I suspect vestibular organ disturbance plays a major role.

2) Visual disturbance: In visually sensitive people, motion detection systems are thrown off by seeing the moving blade shadows on the landscape (which is supposed to be stationary), or by the flickering of sunlight inside as blade shadows cross windows. Two subjects, both adult women prone to vertigo at baseline, were sensitive to the visual channel. They developed severe headaches when exposed to the moving shadows of turbine blades.

3) Somato-sensory disturbance: Abnormal vibration of the ground or floor may send abnormal motion and position signals to brain balance centers via the stretch receptors in muscles and joints of the legs. Several subjects felt this type of vibration, but I don't know if it played a role in their overall balance-related disturbance. I am not sure if this is an important channel.

4) Visceral graviceptor disturbance: This involves the newly discovered fourth channel of motion and position detection—the *visceral graviceptors*, or stretch and pressure receptors in the internal organs of the chest and abdomen. This is the balance channel many physicians are not aware of, since we were all taught in medical school that only three senses feed into balance.

Visceral graviceptors are based on stretch and pressure receptors in and around internal organs. These receptors can let your brain know you're upside down, for example, by detecting that the body's blood mass has shifted from the legs to the chest. They do this by detecting that the large blood vessels in the chest are stretched or have greater mass, or by comparing the pressure of blood inside organs or blood vessels at higher and lower locations in the body. This is thought to be a reason why astronauts orbiting the earth, in what is called "microgravity," can have the sensation they're upside down. Blood vessels in the legs are stronger and stiffer because, in full earth gravity, they have to resist the tendency of the blood to pool at the bottom (in the feet and legs). When gravity is no longer pulling blood to the feet, this natural vascular tone squeezes it all back up into the chest. In gravity, this would only happen if a person was upside down, so this is how the brain interprets this redistribution of blood.

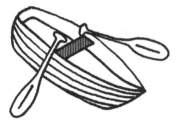

There are suggestions in the balance literature that visceral graviceptors play an important role in car-sickness and seasickness, by being the detectors for unusual up-and-down movements at odds with what the rest of the balance system is saying. It helps in seasickness, for instance, to stand up and look out at the horizon. This brings information from the eyes and stretch receptors in legs in line with the vestibular and visceral motion signals. It also helps you damp with your legs the up-and-down movements your insides are feeling.

The internal graviceptors provide a potential link between the sensations of quivering or pulsation in the chest and the rest of the symptoms of VVVD (*Visceral Vibratory Vestibular Disturbance*), by feeding information about pressure and stretch in the chest directly into the vestibular system. Balaban documents these neural linkages (see below). An alternative, suggested by Dr. Owen Black (a neurotologist), is that pressure changes in the chest may cause changes in the pressure of fluid around the brain (which is known to happen), which may in turn cause pressure inequalities (and thus vestibular symptoms) in the inner ears of people with certain inner-ear problems.

The VVVD story also involves remembering how the chest is a receptor for air pressure fluctuations (described above on pp. 213–14). Every form of sound in air, from low frequency to high frequency, consists of strings of air pressure pulses. When we breathe, our airways and lungs, which fill most of the chest, are open to the air. Sound pressure waves can easily enter and can set this elastic and mobile system moving with very little energy.

The broader role of the stretch and pressure receptors in and around internal organs may in fact be physiologic homeostasis—detecting speed, size, pressure, and flow in one's own heartbeat and breathing, for example, and keeping the brain informed of moment-to-moment status. Pressure detection in the chest is important in the regulation of breathing, since we breathe in by creating negative pressure in the chest, and out by creating positive pressure. Vibration detection may also be critical for monitoring flow in airways or blood vessels. We are very sensitive to (and easily alarmed by) any alterations in the pressure it takes to breathe in or out. I think this is why many subjects in this study felt they couldn't breathe normally when subjected to air pressure pulsations from the turbines: the pulsations triggered the same receptors for pressure and flow as normal breathing, but at the wrong time in the breathing cycle or to an abnormal degree.

Now that we've covered the ways in which wind turbines may cause disturbed balance signaling in susceptible people, let's talk about how we get from disturbed vestibular signaling to some of the less likely-sounding parts of Wind Turbine Syndrome: panic attacks and trouble thinking and remembering.

First, the balance system in the brain is neurologically tied to fear and anxiety.

Back to the fish—to the beginning of the vestibular system. Fish with simple hearing systems, like teleosts, detect nearby movements in the water with their vestibular organs. They use that information to find prey or avoid becoming prey. It makes sense that a system with a critical role in escaping predation would be hardwired into the brain's networks for fear and alerting—for fast escapes. Think too about all those stories of animals detecting and fleeing earthquakes, tsunamis, incipient volcanoes, and ice breakup—things that rumble or make low frequency noise and vibration—long before human beings become aware of them. Detection of this kind of signal is also tied to fear responses: the animals flee.

Dr. Carey Balaban, a brain researcher, studies the brain cell linkages between balance and brain centers controlling anxiety and fear, and between balance, autonomic responses (such as high heart rate, sweating, nausea, etc.), and aversive learning (nausea leading to avoidance). Disordered balance signals feed directly into fear, anxiety, and rapid physical responses, both autonomic (the internal fight-or-flight reaction) and muscular (rapid corrective movement of trunk and limbs). Balaban shows the actual nerve networks mediating these communications in the brain.

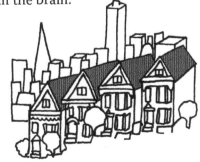

Balaban illustrates with a story. Imagine you're stopped in your car on a hill (facing uphill). Say, San Francisco. Out of the corner of your eye you see the truck next to you start to inch forward. This immediately gives you the impression you're starting to slip backwards! You panic! You jam your foot on the brake! The fear subsides as you realize you are in fact . . . not moving.

Balaban's story underscores that when you sense you're not stable in space—you're going to fall, you're moving when you don't expect it—it grabs all your attention, immediately, with alerting and fear. If the sensation of unexpected movement goes on over a long time, as in vertigo, the sense of fear can also become chronic.

Studies by psychiatrists and balance specialists show how the links between anxiety and balance problems play out clinically and in real life. A mild form of balance disorder is called *space and motion discomfort*, in which people feel uncomfortable or dizzy in situations like supermarket aisles, looking up at tall buildings, closing their eyes in the shower, leaning far back in a chair, driving through tunnels, riding in an elevator, or reading in the car. These people also have abnormalities on balance testing. It's usually a central balance problem, meaning the brain has difficulty integrating all the different signals coming into the balance system, and deciding which ones to ignore if they don't match.

Space and motion discomfort is common in people with migraine disorders. So are dizziness, vertigo (spinning dizziness), and motion sickness. Balance testing tends to be abnormal in people with migraine disorder compared to people who get other kinds of headaches, especially if the migraine patient is one who gets dizziness or vertigo. The balance problems in migraine disorder, incidentally, are sometimes based in the inner-ear vestibular organs and sometimes in the brain.

Anxiety problems are also associated with migraine, sharing a common thread in the serotonin systems of the brain. *Space and motion discomfort* is common in people with anxiety disorders.

Balance testing shows that anxiety patients have higher vestibular (inner ear) sensitivity than people without anxiety problems. When balance testing is done in people diagnosed with panic attacks or agoraphobia (fear of leaving the house), a high number are found to have abnormalities of vestibular (inner ear) function—more than 80% in some studies. This is especially true if the people have episodes of dizziness between panic attacks.

In sum, *there is a robust clinical and experimental literature supporting a biological connection between balance disturbance and anxiety, and between balance problems and panic attacks.* Thus it makes eminent clinical sense that *disturbing a person's balance system can lead to fear, alerting, and panic,* including physical symptoms like fast heartbeat.

Next, thinking and memory. Current research demonstrates that these, too, depend on coherent vestibular signaling. If you don't know which way is up, literally, at all times, your brain can't figure out a multitude of things related to position in space. This can be:

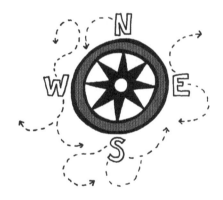

1) *position in real space*, like

    a) remembering how to get somewhere or
    b) figuring out how to put something together, or

2) *position in conceptual space*, like

    a) the distance between two numbers or

b) the position of events in time or

c) the categorization of objects in memory

Neuroscientists have recently shown that nerves from the vestibular system follow a direct, two-neuron path to the hippocampus, a brain structure critical for memory in general and spatial learning in particular. People with no inner-ear input to the brain at all (the nerves having been cut years before to remove tumors) cannot do experimental tasks involving navigation and spatial memory, and their hippocampi (plural of hippocampus) are smaller than normal. (Conversely, taxicab drivers in London have extra-large hippocampi, the size depending on how many years they have been driving and storing in their brains their personal map data of locations, shortcuts, and one-way streets.)

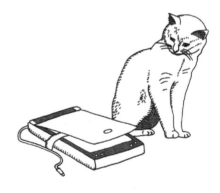

Functional MRI and PET scans (PET scans don't scan your pet, just as CAT scans don't scan your kitty; see Abbreviations, p. 257) now allow researchers to see which parts of the brain are used for different tasks by awake humans while they are doing things. Stimulating the vestibular (inner-ear balance) system lights up many areas in the brain, including those used for mental representations of space and mathematical thinking.

If the vestibular input is distorted (for example, by putting ice water in one ear), people make more mistakes in purely mental spatial tasks like imagining a certain object in detail or imagining rotating it. These people were sitting still when they were tested, eyes closed, just thinking, not trying to keep their balance or having to judge where they were in space at all. Nonetheless, when signals came from one inner ear indicating movement—signals out of whack with all the other signals their balance centers were receiving—they remembered the objects less accurately and made mistakes when imagining them in different positions.

In other words, *disordered signaling from the inner ear degrades both spatial memory and the efficiency and accuracy of spatial thinking.* We call the quality of efficiency and accuracy of thinking *concentration.*

A cluster of brain centers that receive signals from the inner ear (meaning, they become active on functional MRI or PET studies when the vestibular organs are stimulated) are in the parietal ("par-rye-et-al") lobes of the brain. There can be some very weird outcomes if the right-sided parietal centers are lost to a right-sided stroke. Called "hemineglect" (*hemi* = "half" + *neglect* meaning neglect of half the body and half of space), the poor souls so afflicted can have so much unawareness of the left side of space that they can be unaware that their left arm is paralyzed or the left side of their body undressed. Vestibular stimulation, however, temporarily reverses the neglect, so that they become aware of the left side again in a more normal way.

People with hemineglect make certain types of errors on visual search and visual memory tasks, with answers biased away from the left and towards the right sides of images. Left vestibular stimulation corrects or improves performance on these tasks.

Other studies of people with hemineglect let us see what other kinds of mental tasks are "spatialized," meaning, they require the spatial types of thinking done in these right parietal lobe centers linked to the vestibular system. Spatialized thinking includes mathematical operations like forming a mental image of a ruler (lower numbers on the left, higher on the right), and imagining the midpoint between two numbers. It also includes clock representations of time, and spelling at the beginning (left) and ending (right) of words.

Studies of powerful thinkers also show how important spatial thinking is. Great mathematicians think of math in spatial terms (which is efficient, because the actual neural representation of numbers is spatial), and outstanding memorizers use spatially oriented strategies.

In summary, *many things we do with our brains rely on spatial thinking or memory.* Spatial thinking in turn requires vestibular input in good order: literally, we need to know which way is up to know where anything is in physical or conceptual space. Reduction or distortion of vestibular neural signals knocks spatial thinking off balance, so to speak, rendering it less efficient and less accurate.

Now think about the specific tasks my study subjects had trouble with—what they spontaneously told me about themselves and their children, along the lines of:

a) "I can't believe I can't manage something this simple anymore!"

b) "He (my child) knew how to do this, and now he can't do it at all and gets really mad and frustrated when I make him keep trying!"

Below, the letter and number refers to the person's CASE HISTORIES table. I have added a description of the *spatial quality* of each task in italics:

A1 Remembering what he had come to get when he arrived at a store. *Spatial memory for the image of what he was searching for.*

B2 Remembering a series of errands and things to get in town. *Spatial memory for the objects and places to get them, spatial calculation of the most efficient path and order.*

C1, D1, G3 Reading. *Conversion of spatial input (words on page) to language and then to concepts and imagery (which are also spatial). There is also direct vestibular control of eye movements.*

C2, G2 Multitasking in kitchen and household. *Having an internal map of the locations and timing of multiple things at once, inserting tasks and events into the map and not losing awareness of them when out of sight.*

C7 Math—lost skills and forgot math facts. *Spatial representation of numbers and number relationships.*

E2 Spelling, writing. *Putting letters in the right order so the word looks right; changing language into a visual representation.*

F2 Assembling furniture. *Being able to convert written instructions or diagrams to a three-dimensional mental representation of what she was supposed to do with the pieces.*

F2 Following the steps in a simple recipe. *Picturing and ordering the steps in mind from the written instructions.*

F2 Following the plot of a TV mystery. *Noticing, remembering, and putting together visual clues.*

F3 Did worse than in the past on national exams. *Outstanding memorizers use spatial strategies, as described above.*

H3 Reading, spelling, math. *All of these have significant spatial components.*

I1 Professional landscaping and gardening—loss of concentration. *Planning and arranging things in space, remembering where he put down a tool, judging if something he's building is turning out right and how to fix it, planning the steps of tasks efficiently in time and space, not forgetting steps.*

J1 Paying bills. *Mathematics, memory for objects and services purchased, mental calculation of future needs.*

Each problematic task shows spatial thinking full of errors and inefficiencies, and people enormously frustrated over normal, common-sense things they suddenly can't do efficiently. ("Common sense" has a big spatial thinking component, too.) Early school learning is also thrown off, and reading and certain higher memory and problem-solving skills in adults.

Interference of noise with reading and children's learning is not a new discovery. There is an extensive literature on it. In brief, environmental noise such as airport or traffic noise makes children learn to read more slowly. In these studies, large numbers of children were studied in 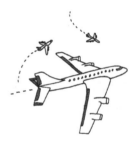 carefully controlled exposed and non-exposed groups, by choosing school districts at different locations relative to airports. Children were exposed to the extra noise both in school and at home.

In one study, a city closed an old airport and built a new one, and researchers had the opportunity to follow the reading skills of both sets of children over time. The ones living near the airport that closed showed improvements in their reading. The ones near the new airport showed slower learning after planes started flying in and out.

One study looked at children living in an apartment building next to a busy highway. Those on the higher floors, where it was quieter, had better reading scores and better ability to tell word sounds apart.

The effects of noise on reading ability go beyond the distracting effects of noise, and are linked to problems with language processing—like differentiating between language sounds—in noisy environments.

Noise has been shown to affect thinking in adults, too, in other settings and at loudness levels nowhere near the levels that harm hearing. In one study, industrial workers worked on psychological tests while exposed to 50 dBA broadband noise (like white or machine noise) with or without low frequency components. The noise with low frequency components interfered with test performance more than the noise without low frequencies, especially in individuals who rated themselves as sensitive to low frequency noise. Neither type of noise was considered more annoying than the other, nor did subjects become accustomed or sensitized to the noise.

Many environmental noise studies have examined effects of nighttime community noise on sleep, stress hormone (adrenaline and cortisol) levels, blood pressure, and cardiovascular risk factors. There are positive, significant associations between noise and each of these factors: noise exposure increases stress hormone output, blood pressure, and general cardiovascular risk. High stress hormone levels elevate blood sugar and increase blood pressure, two elements of cardiovascular risk.

Noise at night can significantly disturb sleep even when the person does not remember waking up. Since the sorting and daily storage of memories occurs during sleep (especially during REM or rapid eye movement sleep), sleep disturbance by noise—even without known awakening—degrades memory and learning. Memory and learning are also degraded by long-term elevated cortisol levels in chronically stressed people, probably by reducing the survival rate of new hippocampal memory cells.

In children, exposure to nighttime noise with low frequency components (rumbling/vibrating noise from trucks passing close to the outside walls of their houses) provokes more stress hormone production early in the night than does exposure to car traffic noise without the trucks.

Interestingly, the levels of noise that disturb sleep are quite low. Noise events of 32 dBA cause people to move in sleep, showing a low level of arousal. Noise events of 35 dBA cause arousals that can be seen on a brain wave study (EEG). Conscious awakenings occur at noise events of 42 dBA. This is why the World Health Organization (WHO) recommends 30 dBA as an acceptable indoor nighttime noise level.

I don't present noise analyses in this paper—something that clearly needs to be done, but requires resources I didn't have—but I find that published descriptions of people's experiences in documented low frequency noise investigations are very similar to what my study subjects noticed and described to me. If you haven't already done so, I recommend you read the section of the REPORT FOR CLINICIANS called "Low frequency noise" (p. 104).

Dr. Birgitta Berglund (a dean of community noise studies and lead editor of the 1999 World Health Organization *Guidelines for Community Noise*) describes why she thinks many of the adverse effects of community noise in general are due to its low frequency components. She notes how low frequency noise travels farther than higher frequency noise without losing its power, travels through walls and hearing protectors, rattles objects, sets up vibrations and resonances in the human body, and is linked to motion sickness even when vibration is not present. Low frequency noise makes it hard to distinguish sounds at higher frequencies, like speech sounds. Noise with low frequency components is experienced as louder and more annoying than noise at the same dBA level without low frequency components.

It's important to remember that the term "annoyance" in community noise surveys is used as a shorthand for a variety of negative reactions—some of them severe. "Apart from 'annoyance,'" states the WHO, "people...exposed to community noise...report anger, disappointment, dissatisfaction, withdrawal, helplessness, depression, anxiety, distraction, agitation, or exhaustion."

In the REPORT FOR CLINICIANS, I quote as well several other small studies of situations wherein people were exposed to documented low frequency noise. For instance, the symptoms felt by healthy young men while exposed to high amplitude low frequency noise for only 2–3 minutes, in a NASA test facility in the 1960s, included fatigue, reduced efficiency at performing tasks, tickling in the ear, chest vibrations, and a feeling of fullness in the throat—all symptoms I heard about from my study's participants.

Indeed a case report from Germany in 1996 may well be Wind Turbine Syndrome, since the source of the low frequency noise (actually infrasound, below 10 Hz) was never identified. It's an especially interesting story. The couple's symptoms and the intensity of noise below 10 Hz both varied with the wind and weather, and were worse in winter. Their symptoms were:

a)   sleep disturbance
b)   headache

c) ear pressure

d) not feeling well in a general way

e) decreased ability/efficiency in doing things

f) chest symptoms described as shortness of breath and a tingling/crawling sensation

Symptoms occurred when the sound pressure level at 1 Hz was 65 dB, well below the couple's own hearing thresholds measured in a sound lab. All the frequencies responsible for the symptoms, which were all below 10 Hz, had sound pressure levels below 80 dB.

We now know that sound levels near turbines easily fall within these ranges, as measured by a Dutch physicist several years ago.

The 1996 German case, above, and another series of cases, also by German noise control engineers (see REPORT FOR CLINICIANS, pp. 106–8), both emphasize *how the symptoms and the degree to which the people were bothered increased over time after they moved into the home or apartment with low frequency noise.* They did not get used to the noise. In fact, the opposite: they became sensitized to it over time. At first it wasn't so bad, but it grew worse and worse.

My study subjects said the same thing, as they compared turbine noise to other types of noise, like traffic, that they easily got used to. Many said that wind turbine noise would not sound loud to people who did not live with it,[2] but several also mentioned visitors being

---

[2] An interesting instance of this came before the European Court of Human Rights on February 26, 2008, in the case of Lars and Astrid Fägerskiöld v Sweden (Application No.: 00037664/04). The plaintiffs cited Article 8 of the Convention and Article 1 of Protocol No. 1 to the Convention. The following passages are taken from the court brief.

"According to the applicants, the wind turbine emitted a constant, pulsating noise and, sometimes, light effects which *they found very disturbing and intrusive.* For these reasons and because they considered that the new wind turbine had been

bothered while spending only one night. When they moved away from their turbine-exposed homes, all the families moved into towns and villages with more traffic noise, but no risk of turbines being built next door.

Hence, glib claims that "you will get used to wind turbine noise" are contradicted both by people who struggle to live with it and by clinical evidence.

Both German case studies focused on the ability of low frequency noise, with its long wavelengths, to pass through walls and then reverberate or set up resonances inside rooms. The authors of the case series measured the difference in low frequency noise intensity near walls and away from walls, picking up nodes of higher intensity away from walls, like a standing wave in a stream.

---

erected much too close to their property, and without them having been consulted in advance, they complained about it in a letter to the municipality" (emphasis added).

"The applicants appealed to the County Administrative Court (länsrätten) of the County of Östergötland, maintaining their claims. In particular, *they emphasised that the wind turbine was a serious nuisance* and that the Environmental Committee had made an incorrect evaluation of the matter and several formal errors in its handling of the case. Moreover, they stated that the municipality had refused to carry out an impartial noise investigation despite requests from several of the concerned parties" (emphasis added).

"On 14 April 1999, after having visited the applicants' property, the County Administrative Board rejected their appeal.... *It found from its visit to the applicants' property that the wind turbine created certain sound effects which could be considered disturbing but which were not serious enough to justify dismantling the turbine*. In this respect, it noted that the measured noise levels did not reach the maximum recommended level of 40 dB" (emphasis added).

"On 14 July 2000, after having visited the applicants' property and held an oral hearing, the County Administrative Court rejected the appeal. It found that the Environment Committee's decision had been lawful and that, *although some sound effects from the wind turbine could be observed on the applicants' property, the disturbance had to be considered tolerable*" (emphasis added).

The court dismissed the claim.

In my study, Mr. and Mrs. G (G1 and G2) both identified a spot in one room where they got symptoms, a feeling of internal vibration for Mrs. G and the beginnings of nausea for her husband. They could not feel any vibrations with their hands if they touched walls or furniture. I think this was one of those places where the low frequency sound (air pressure) waves overlapped in such a way, as they bounced around the room, that they made a stable spot or standing wave of increased intensity.

Swedish researchers verified in a survey study of hundreds of households that the amount of noise needed to cause severe annoyance is much lower for a wind turbine than for road traffic, airplanes, or trains (see pp. 112–13 in REPORT FOR CLINICIANS). "Amount of noise" was modeled or calculated (rather than measured) based on distance from turbines and turbine power. Noise was modeled in dBA (which doesn't take into account low frequency components even if they are present) and averaged over time.

Results showed that 15% of people were highly annoyed at 38 dBA from wind turbines, compared to 57 dBA for aircraft, 63 dBA for road traffic, and 70 dBA for trains. By the time the wind turbine noise level reached 41 dBA, 35% of people were highly annoyed. Sixteen percent reported sleep disturbance over 35 dBA of outdoor turbine noise.

When these researchers interviewed some of the people they had surveyed, to go into more depth, they found the same sorts of problems I encountered in my study, including people who had moved out of their homes because of the noise or rebuilt their homes to try to exclude the noise. Some reported feeling invaded or violated by turbine noise, being sensitive to blade motion as well as noise, and loss of their ability to rest and feel restored at home.

From this one can reasonably conclude that, for wind turbines, perhaps unlike other sources of noise, *community standards allowing 45–55 dBA outside neighboring homes are asking for trouble.* Wind turbine noise is different and more problematic (perhaps because of the low frequencies excluded by dBA measurements), so the same numerical standards do not apply.

In 2007, Pedersen joined with van den Berg, a Dutch physicist, to further study annoyance around wind turbines, this time in the Netherlands. They found similar results for annoyance at (modeled) wind turbine noise compared to other types of noise. In the Dutch survey results, however, a new element has been quietly introduced into the equation. The owners of turbines lived the closest to turbines, *they benefited economically, and they were able to turn the turbines off if they or their neighbors were troubled by the noise*—a critical difference from other countries. If turbines were getting switched off when people were going nuts from noise in Canada, the USA, the UK, Ireland, or Italy, I would not be writing this report.

Van den Berg and Pedersen also claim to have studied health relative to wind turbine noise—except their attempt to do so was flawed to the point of being valueless. The proof is in plain sight in their reported results. Their mail-in survey only asked two questions about health. (Questions about sleep were separate.) One asked about all chronic disease, past and present, in one question. The answers show bias—meaning the survey (either because of the way people were chosen or the way the questions drew information out of them) failed to get an accurate picture of the number of people with these chronic diseases in the study population. We know this because, for at least two of the chronic conditions asked about, migraine and tinnitus, the numbers were much lower than the real population prevalences as known from many, well-constructed studies.

Yet the authors charge ahead and use their data set as if it were valid, to test a hypothesis that is equally ill-considered—that health effects, if present, would show up as more chronic disease (any chronic disease under the sun) closer to turbines than up to a mere 2.1 km (1.3 miles) away. They expect to prove or disprove this with a small set of vague survey results that could not even capture 20% of the migraine disorder present in the population. As a clinician (I believe neither van den Berg nor Pedersen is one), I can say categorically that the kinds of studies that can show the effect of noise on chronic health conditions have huge data sets and a huge study population (or study samples), and the information on the chronic illness (which is always cardiovascular disease or stress hormone production, when noise and health are studied) is carefully defined in subjects and controls. You simply can't approach this question with van den Berg's and Pedersen's kind of data. The juxtaposition of the hypothesis, above, with their method of data collection don't go together. Clinically speaking, their study has no merit.

Let me be emphatic. *You can't start with an implausible hypothesis or a flawed data set and get a result that means anything.* Where health is concerned, van den Berg and Pedersen don't grasp this. They crunch lots of numbers, but are not realistic about the limitations of their health data set and how these restrict the conclusions they can draw.

The second of the two health questions, a list of possible "current symptoms," is a weird mish-mash of physical and psychological symptoms with a few plain old "feeling words" thrown in. Their question yielded virtually no useful information. They mention this question exactly once in their analysis, to remark that survey respondents who did not benefit economically reported more health symptoms than those who benefited, and that this difference could have been due to the systematic age difference between those who benefited and those who did not (who were older).

Despite health being inadequately sampled in this study, van den Berg and Pedersen nonetheless draw conclusions that are interpreted popularly as evidence against health effects by wind turbines. Consider this statement from their summary: "There is no indication that the sound from wind turbines had an effect on respondents' health, except for the interruption of sleep" (p. ii). Though soft-pedaled by the authors, sleep interruption is in fact of enormous significance to health. Over and above the sleep issue, they are remiss in failing to acknowledge that their study did not have the power to detect other health effects.

In sum, van den Berg and Pedersen could have better captured the survey's (limited) health results had they written, "Sleep disturbance or interruption, an effect of profound importance to health, was correlated with turbine noise levels. Unfortunately, the survey could not effectively address other health questions due to bias introduced at the level of data collection. An important finding is the possibility of biased responses from respondents benefiting economically from turbines, yet it is equally possible that turbine owners are in the habit of turning turbines off at critical times, thus avoiding both annoyance and sleep disturbance."

Recommendations

George Kamperman and Rick James, two independent American noise control engineers with decades of experience working with industrial noise and communities, recommend a noise standard based on quietest background ambient noise, using C-weighted as well as A-weighted measurements so that the low frequency components are controlled. Their specific recommendations—for how noise measurements should be done and how procedures should be spelled out in a local ordinance—were presented at the annual conference of the Institute of Noise Control Engineering/USA in 2008 and are posted on the Wind Turbine Syndrome website at www.windturbinesyndrome.com/?p=925. An important outcome of Kamperman and James's method is that as turbines get larger, setbacks will have to be greater.

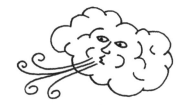

The simple answer is: *Keep wind turbines at least 2 km (1¼ miles) away on the flat, and 3.2 km (2 miles) in mountains. These are minimum distances. Kamperman and James's methods will likely recommend larger setbacks, especially in rural areas that are very quiet at baseline.* Second, all wind turbine ordinances should hold developers responsible for a full price (pre-turbine) buyout of any family whose lives are ruined by turbines—to prod developers to follow realistic health-based rules and prevent the extreme economic loss of home abandonment.

A 2 km setback would have prevented this:[3]

> My husband is seeing a doctor for depression. I have a daughter who is seeing a specialist for serious stomach problems. I have had endless sleepless nights since the wind turbines went up. I constantly have feelings of anxiety. My children have complained of headaches and not sleeping well.
>
> Let me ask you, What would you do?

What would I do? I admit I'd be driven into doing what she has done:

---

[3] Personal communication, April 6, 2009.

I have been forced to make a decision I never thought I'd have to make. My husband and I have decided to walk away from our property. I can't stand it here for another day. I can't leave soon enough. You may be able to put turbines up behind our home, but that doesn't mean I am going to do nothing when it affects my family's health and my animals' well-being.

It's too late for me to take any more chances. I have kids I need to get through college. I don't know how I'll do it. I just know it's not good to live in this house any more. This property I once loved and was so proud to own is of no use to me.

I have worked 60 hours a week for years, only to find myself with nothing. But my health as well as my family's cannot be sacrificed.

So, as you read this, I do not know where we are going to live, but I do know it won't be under a wind turbine or anywhere near one. The safest bet would be to find a house right next door to the people who determine these setbacks, because no matter what they decide, it seems they are never the people affected.

She closed her letter: "Ann Wirtz, N11957 Highway YY, Oakfield, Wisconsin 53065 (temporarily)."

Consider the pain of that final word. *Temporarily.* In parentheses. Like quiet despair. "The heaviness of life," offered Rilke, "is heavier even than the weight of things."[4]

---

[4] Rilke, Rainer Maria. 1981. "The Neighbor." *Selected Poems of Rainer Maria Rilke: A Translation from the German and Commentary by Robert Bly.* Harper & Row, New York, p. 93.

Abbreviations

χ^2	chi-squared statistic or test
ACL	anterior cruciate ligament
BP	blood pressure
CAT	computerized axial tomography
dB	decibels
dBA	decibels measured with an A-weighted filter
dBC	decibels measured with a C-weighted filter
CSF	cerebrospinal fluid
EEG	electroencephalogram
EH	endolymphatic hydrops
ft	feet
GER	gastroesophageal reflux
GI	gastrointestinal
h/o	history of
Hz	Hertz (frequency in per second or sec^{-1})
INCE	Institute of Noise Control Engineering
INR	international normalized ratio of prothrombin times (see GLOSSARY: anticoagulation)
kHz	kiloHertz (1000 Hz)
km	kilometers (1000 m)
m	meters
mcg	micrograms
mi	miles
MI	myocardial infarction
MRA	magnetic resonance angiography
MRI	magnetic resonance imaging
MW	megawatts
N/A	not applicable
OTC	over-the-counter (non-prescription)
OVEMP	ocular vestibular evoked myogenic potential

p	when used in the context of a statistical test, p means probability that the compared distributions are no different from each other
P.E.	professional engineer
PE	pressure equalization
PET	positron emission tomography
PTSD	post-traumatic stress disorder
TENS	transcutaneous electrical nerve stimulation
URI	upper respiratory infection (viral cold)
VAD	vibroacoustic disease
VEMP	vestibular evoked myogenic potential
VVVD	Visceral Vibratory Vestibular Disturbance
WHO	World Health Organization
WTS	Wind Turbine Syndrome

Glossary

A-weighting network: an electronic filter that reduces the contribution of low frequencies to a sound measurement; see pp. 36–38, 214–15.

Acute gastrointestinal infection: nausea, vomiting, abdominal pain, and diarrhea, generally self-limited and caused by a viral infection of the gastrointestinal tract.

Agoraphobia: an abnormal fear of leaving the house.

Air-conducted sound: sound that travels through the air and reaches the inner ear by way of the external auditory canal, tympanic membrane (eardrum) and the three ossicles of the middle ear. See *bone-conducted sound*.

Airways: trachea, bronchi, and bronchioles, the tubular structures through which air passes to reach the air sacs or alveoli of the lungs.

Amaurosis fugax: temporary loss of vision in one eye.

Analgesic: pain medication.

Anticoagulation: use of medications such as heparin or warfarin to decrease the tendency of the blood to clot. Higher INR (international normalized ratio of prothrombin time) values, used in the monitoring of warfarin administration, indicate slower or less effective clotting.

Antihypertensive: blood pressure medication.

Anxiolytic: anti-anxiety medication.

Arthralgia: joint pain without objective signs of inflammation (see *arthritis*).

Arthritis: pain and/or stiffness in joints with accompanying objective signs of inflammation, such as redness or swelling.

Asthma: intermittent and reversible respiratory difficulty caused by partial obstruction of small airways by inflammation/swelling and constriction of smooth muscle around the airways. Asthma attacks may be provoked by any kind of respiratory infection, allergic exposures, or irritant exposures.

Ataxia, ataxic: in reference to gait, unsteady on feet, difficulty with balance or coordination in walking, or difficulty maintaining posture, for neurologic reasons.

Atrial fibrillation: an abnormal heart rhythm in which the small chambers do not pump rhythmically, but instead vibrate erratically, placing patients at risk for stroke from blood clots that can form inside the heart.

Autonomic nervous system: the involuntary part of the nervous system that regulates automatic body functions such as heart rate, blood pressure, gastrointestinal function, sweating, glandular output, pupillary reflexes, airway smooth muscle tone, and others. The autonomic system includes sensory receptors (for afferent signals or input to the central nervous system) and effector neurons (for efferent signals or output to organs). It consists of opposing sympathetic and parasympathetic networks. Sympathetic stimulation speeds the heart and readies the body for optimal "fight or flight" activity. Parasympathetic stimulation slows the heart, lowers blood pressure, and facilitates digestion.

Baroreceptors: pressure detectors, as in blood vessels or lungs.

Basilar migraine: migraine with auras representing brainstem effects, including vertigo, tinnitus, fluctuations in level of consciousness, and temporary motor deficits.

Bilateral: on both sides of the body.

Binaural processing: brain integration of hearing signals from both ears.

Bone-conducted sound: sound or vibratory stimulus reaching the inner ear via direct solid-to-solid and solid-to-fluid transmission, without passing through or utilizing the tympanic membrane or middle ear ossicles. It is created by placing a vibrating object against the skin over a skull bone, typically the mastoid process immediately behind the ear. See *air-conducted sound*.

Bronchodilator: medication used to relax airway smooth muscle in the treatment of asthma, usually inhaled.

C-weighting network: an electronic filter that reduces the contribution of very low frequencies to a sound measurement, but less so than an A-weighting network; see pp. 36–38, 214–215.

Caloric test: a test of semicircular canal function and the vestibulo-ocular response. In the caloric response to ice water in the external auditory canal, thermal convection induces fluid movement within the horizontal semicircular canal, creating an illusion of head movement that is reflected in eye movement via the vestibulo-ocular reflex.

Cardiac arrhythmia or dysrhythmia: specific types of irregular heartbeat, often occurring episodically.

Catecholamine: a class of biochemicals that function as neurotransmitters in the brain and as hormones produced by the sympathetic part of the autonomic nervous system, such as epinephrine (adrenaline), norepinephrine, and dopamine.

Central: occurring in the brain (central nervous system), as opposed to a peripheral neural receptor, effector, or organ. For example, central processing, central origin, central dysfunction.

Cerebellum, cerebellar: a posterior/inferior portion of the brain with important functions in coordination and integration of movement.

Cerebrospinal fluid: clear fluid that circulates from fluid spaces (lateral ventricles) in the brain, where it is produced, through the other ventricles and around the brain and spinal cord.

Chemotherapy: in this report, refers specifically to medications given for cancer treatment.

Cilium, cilia: actively motile, hair-like projections from epithelial cell surfaces in the airways and Eustachian tubes that beat in synchrony to move mucus out of these moist, air-filled spaces, towards the pharynx.

Circadian rhythm: a daily physiologic cycle, such as sleep and wakefulness or the peaks and troughs of cortisol secretion.

Cochlea: spiral-shaped sensory organ of hearing, part of the inner-ear membranous labyrinth. See pp. 200–201.

Collagen: a protein which is the chief substance of connective tissue, cartilage, tendons, etc.

Concussion: mild brain injury produced by impact to the head resulting in brief unconsciousness, disorientation, or memory problem.

Conductive hearing loss: hearing loss due to problems in the outer ear, tympanic membrane, or middle ear.

Coronary artery disease: partial obstruction or narrowing of the small arteries that supply the heart muscle.

Cortex, cortical: the outer cellular layers of the two cerebral hemispheres of the brain.

Cortisol: a major natural glucocorticoid hormone produced by the adrenal cortex in a regular daily rhythm and in response to stress, which exerts diverse effects on tissues and metabolic processes throughout the body.

Cranial vault: the space in the skull that contains the brain.

Diaphragm: the dome-shaped sheet of skeletal muscle that separates the thoracic (chest) and abdominal cavities and enables breathing.

Dysfunction: malfunction or poor functioning.

Elastin: an elastic connective tissue protein, which gives elasticity to certain structures, such as arterial walls.

Electroencephalogram (EEG): a recording of brain waves monitored in a specific fashion, used in studies of seizure disorder and sleep.

Endolymphatic hydrops (EH): a condition of distorted fluid and pressure relationships between the endolymph and perilymph, which are the two fluid compartments in the inner ear. This causes erratic and distorted balance and, often, hearing signals to be sent to the brain. Meniere's disease and perilymphatic fistula are examples of conditions with endolymphatic hydrops.

Epithelial basement membrane: a thin layer of extracellular proteins and mucopolysaccharides that lies at the base of and supports the layers of cells comprising an epithelium, such as the linings of airways, mouth, esophagus, intestine, pleura, etc.

Eustachian tube: a tube that connects the middle ear with the nasopharynx, or upper part of the throat behind the nose. It allows equalization of air pressure on either side of the tympanic membrane.

Fibromyalgia: a condition of chronic pain of unclear origin, in muscles, ligaments, and tendons, without inflammation.

Gastritis: inflammation of the lining of the stomach causing pain and nausea.

Gastroesophageal reflux (GER): reflux or intrusion of acidic stomach contents into the esophagus; heartburn.

Gastrointestinal (GI) tract: stomach, small intestine, and colon or large intestine.

Glucose instability: in diabetes, fluctuating blood sugar levels that go too high or too low.

Glucosuria: glucose in urine, a sign of poor diabetic control.

Graviceptors: neural detectors of gravity and acceleration; see pp. 73–74, 234–35.

Great vessels: the large arteries and veins immediately around the heart, including the aorta, pulmonary artery, pulmonary veins, and superior and inferior vena cavae.

Hair cells: mechanoreceptive cells in the inner-ear labyrinthine organs (cochlea, semicircular canals, utricle, and saccule). These cells send neural signals when mechanically perturbed or bent. Local properties of parts of the membranous labyrinth control how the hair cells are perturbed.

Hippocampus: a brain region in the medial temporal lobe critical to spatial navigation and formation of new episodic memories.

Hyperacusis: oversensitivity to sound, with normal sounds seeming painfully loud.

Hypertension: high blood pressure.

Hypopharynx: the lower part of the throat, just above the larynx (vocal cords).

Immissions: in acoustics, sound from the point of view of the person or location receiving the sound. *Emissions* in this context refers to the sound as it leaves the source.

In utero: in the uterus during pregnancy.

Infrasonic: sound frequency below hearing range, generally considered to be 20 Hz or less.

Irritable bowel syndrome: recurrent episodes of abdominal pain and diarrhea, often with alternating periods of constipation, without any pathologic or inflammatory changes in the gastrointestinal tract.

Labyrinthine organs, membranous labyrinth: the inner-ear organs, including the cochlea, utricle, saccule, and semicircular canals. See *otolith organs* and *semicircular canals*, and pp. 200–201.

Lower respiratory infection: bronchitis, pneumonia, or pneumonia with pleural effusion (pleurisy).

Lupus: systemic lupus erythematosus, a systemic inflammatory or autoimmune disease affecting the skin, joints, gastrointestinal tract, kidney, blood, and brain.

Macula: in the otolith organs (utricle and saccule), the patch of sensory hair cells plus superimposed mass of otoconia in a protein matrix (sometimes called *macule*). See p. 200.

Magnetic resonance angiography (MRA): a noninvasive imaging method for examining the patency of blood vessels.

Magnetic resonance imaging (MRI): soft-tissue imaging using magnetic fields, providing the most detailed images of living brain structure available. Functional magnetic resonance imaging (fMRI) quantifies blood flow to different brain structures during specific activities.

Malaise: a vague sense of not feeling well.

Mastoid: a bony structure immediately behind the ear that contains air-filled cells connected to the middle ear.

Mediastinum: the central portion of the chest or thorax between the lungs, containing the heart, great vessels, trachea, esophagus, lymph nodes, and other structures.

Mesentery: a fold of membranous tissue encasing and attaching the small intestine and other abdominal organs to the inside of the peritoneal (abdominal) cavity, also supporting blood vessels and nerves to the organs.

Microvilli: hair-like projections from epithelial cell surfaces that increase absorptive surface area, for example, in the small intestine.

Migraine: a hereditary, episodic, neurologic condition generally involving severe headaches that may be preceded by visual or other sensory phenomena such as tingling or numbness (aura), with symptoms of nausea and sensitivity to light and sound commonly accompanying headaches. A headache may be one-sided or pounding. Aura and accompanying symptoms may include vertigo, tinnitus, temporary focal weakness or paralysis, temporary loss of vision, vomiting, or loss of consciousness. Sensory sensitivities and triggers include motion, odors, a wide variety of foods (especially products of fermentation or aging, caffeine, chocolate, and varieties of plants), hormonal state, and sleep deprivation.

Migraineur: a person who gets migraines.

Myocardial infarction (MI): heart attack, or obstructed coronary blood flow leading to death of cardiac muscle.

Near-field sound: sound at distances significantly less than one wavelength, especially applicable to hearing under water (e.g., in fish), where wavelengths of sound are much longer than in air (by a factor of 5 at the same frequency), and for lower sound frequencies (which have longer wavelengths in any medium). Near-field sound detection involves detection of particle movement or bulk flow of the medium, rather than a repetitive pressure fluctuation as for *far-field sound* detection in air, for which the mammalian ear and cochlea are specialized.

Neuroanatomic: referring to the anatomy of neural linkages in the brain.

Neuroendocrine: relating to cells or tissues that release hormones into the blood in response to a neural stimulus.

Night terror: a parasomnia, or sleep disturbance occurring during disordered arousal from the deeper stages of sleep, in which a person (usually a child) may scream, act afraid, say nonsensical things, or get up to do irrational or fearful things, all without memory in the morning.

Nocturia: awakening and getting up repeatedly in the night to urinate.

Nocturnal enuresis: bed-wetting while asleep.

Norepinephrine: a central catecholamine neurotransmitter, sympathetic nervous system neurotransmitter, and vasoactive adrenal medullary hormone.

Nystagmus: a pattern of eye movement indicating a disordered vestibulo-ocular reflex that is often due to disordered vestibular signaling or processing, as in the caloric test.

Orbit: the eye socket or hollow space in the skull that contains the eyeball and its associated structures.

Otitis media: middle-ear infection.

Otoconia: microscopic calcium carbonate stones positioned in a protein matrix over the mechanically sensing hair cells of the mammalian utricle and saccule.

Otolith organs: the utricle and saccule, labyrinthine organs of the inner ear that detect linear acceleration, including gravity, by virtue of microscopic calcium carbonate stones or *otoconia* positioned in a protein matrix over the mechanically sensing hair cells. See pp. 200–201.

Palpitations: irregular or pounding heart at times not expected from activity or exertion.

Panic attack: an episode of sudden intense fear out of proportion to circumstances, which may be accompanied by symptoms of dizziness, sweating, trembling, chest pain, palpitations, and the feeling of not being able to get enough breath.

Parabrachial nucleus: brain center involved in extended vestibular system influence, located in the pons.

Parasomnia: a sleep disturbance occurring during disordered arousal from the deeper stages of sleep, such as sleep walking, sleep talking, and night terrors.

Paresthesia: tingling or "pins and needles" sensation, as when a numb extremity is waking up.

Parkinson's disease: a neurologic degenerative disease involving dopamine-producing neural tracts in the brain and affecting movement and psychiatric status.

Pericardium: the two-layered membranous sac that encloses the heart and the roots of the great vessels, in which the heart beats.

Perilymphatic fistula syndrome: see *endolymphatic hydrops* and pp. 93, 227.

Pharynx: the throat.

Pleura: the outer epithelial surface of the lung and the lining of the thoracic cavity, providing low friction surfaces for lung movement.

Pleurisy: inflammation or infection of pleura, which can accompany pneumonia.

Polyuria: excessive daily volume of urine, a typical sign of high glucose levels in diabetics.

Positron emission tomography (PET): a method of functional imaging that quantifies glucose uptake by different brain regions as a measure of activity.

Posturography: a form of balance testing that is sensitive to the vestibulo-spinal reflexes, including the influence of inner-ear, visual, somatosensory, and central processing on the movements by which a subject remains balanced and upright.

Pressure equalization (PE) tube: a tube inserted through a small, surgically placed hole in the tympanic membrane after removal of middle-ear fluid, to provide aeration.

Proton pump inhibitor: medication used to limit stomach acid production in the treatment of gastroesophageal reflux, gastritis, or ulcer.

Resonance: a property of sound; see pp. 36, 211–14.

Retina, retinal: the light-sensing neural structure at the back of the eye.

Saccule: one of the two otolith organs of the vestibular (balance) organs of the inner ear (also called sacculus).

Scotoma: temporary loss of vision in one part of the visual field.

Semicircular canals: bilateral labyrinthine organs of the inner ear that detect angular acceleration of the head by virtue of fluid shifts deflecting mechanically sensing hair cells. See pp. 200–201 and *caloric test*.

Sensorineural hearing loss: hearing loss due to problems in the inner ear/cochlea, vestibulocochlear nerve (cranial nerve VIII), or brain centers that process sound.

Sequela, sequelae: a pathologic condition that develops from another pathologic condition, such as chronic middle-ear fluid and hearing loss being sequelae of repeated acute ear infections.

Serotonin: a brain and gastrointestinal neurotransmitter.

Serous otitis media: viscous fluid in the middle ear (middle-ear effusion) that may obstruct sound transmission, usually occurring after a series of acute ear infections.

Somatic nervous system: the sensory and motor nervous system from and to the skin, skeletal muscles, and associated tendons and ligaments, whose signals may be consciously perceived and voluntarily modified.

Somatosensory: sensory input from the skin, skeletal muscles, tendons, and ligaments.

Sonic: sound frequency in the range of human hearing.

Syncope, syncopal: fainting caused by low blood flow to brain.

Tachycardia: rapid heartbeat.

Taxon, taxa: a group or groups in the scientific categorization (Linnaean taxonomy) of living things.

Temporal bone: solid bone at the base of the skull, in which the labyrinthine organs lie.

Thalamus: a part of the brain involved in part in relaying sensory information to the cerebral cortex.

Tinnitus: "ringing in the ears," which may be a tonal sound, buzzing, white noise, or other types of sound heard in one or both ears. The sound itself is not present in the outside environment.

Trachea: the large central airway between the larynx (voice box) and the split or bifurcation of the right and left bronchi.

Tympanic membrane: eardrum; the layer of taut, thin tissue that separates the external auditory canal from the middle ear.

Ultrasonic: sound frequency above hearing range, generally considered to be 20,000 Hz or more.

Upper gastrointestinal symptoms: gastroesophageal reflux, gastritis, and/or ulcer.

Utricle: one of the two otolith organs of the vestibular (balance) organs of the inner ear (also called utriculus).

Vasculitis: inflammation of blood vessels, which can cause restriction of blood flow.

Vasoconstriction: constriction of a blood vessel.

Vertigo: the spinning form of dizziness, in which the visual surround seems to move.

Vestibular: pertaining to the balance organs in the inner ear (utricle, saccule, and semicircular canals) or to the integrated balance system in general, as in "vestibular areas of the brain."

Vestibular evoked myogenic potential (VEMP): a vestibular reflex neural response, used clinically and in research to test specifically for otolith function or stimulation. Ocular vestibular evoked myogenic potential (OVEMP) is similar. See pp. 85–86, 203.

Vestibulo-collic reflex: a fast or "short-latency" neural response across a short, three-neuron brain arc from the otolith organs to brainstem vestibular nuclei to brain nuclei controlling the muscles of the neck to neck muscles, whose purpose is immediate, automatic stabilization of the head in response to detected motion.

Vestibulo-ocular reflex: a fast or "short-latency" neural response across a short, three-neuron brain arc from the semicircular canals and otolith organs to brainstem vestibular nuclei to brain nuclei controlling extraocular eye muscles to eye muscles, whose purpose is immediate, automatic compensatory movements of the eyes in response to detected head motion, to stabilize the visual field during movement.

Vestibulo-spinal reflex: like the vestibulo-collic reflex but involving muscles below the neck (along the spinal column and in the legs) to stabilize posture during movement and rapidly correct potential falls.

Vibroacoustic disease (VAD): a type of noise-related illness. See pp. 109–11.

Visceral Vibratory Vestibular Disturbance (VVVD): a sensation of internal quivering, vibration, or pulsation accompanied by agitation, anxiety, alarm, irritability, rapid heartbeat, nausea, and sleep disturbance. See pp. 55–60, 76–79, 224, and 235–36.

Whiplash injury: an injury to the neck (cervical vertebrae) caused by abrupt acceleration or deceleration, as in an automobile accident.

References

Académie nationale de médecine de France. 2006. "Le retentissement du fonctionnement des éoliennes sur la santé de l'homme, le Rapport, ses Annexes et les Recommandations de l'Académie nationale de médecine." 17 pp. www.academie-medecine.fr/sites_thematiques/EOLIENNES/chouard_rapp_14mars_2006.htm.

Ahlbom IC, Cardis E, Green A, Linet M, Savitz D, Swerdlow A; INCIRP (International Commission for Non-Ionizing Radiation Protection) Standing Committee on Epidemiology. 2001. Review of the epidemiologic literature on EMF and health. Environ Health Perspect 109 Suppl 6: 911–33.

Babisch W. 2003. Stress hormones in the research on cardiovascular effects of noise. Noise Health 5(18): 1–11.

Babisch W. 2005. Guest editorial: Noise and health. Environ Health Perspect 113(1): A14–15.

Babisch W, Beule B, Schust M, Kersten N, Ising H. 2005. Traffic noise and risk of myocardial infarction. Epidemiology 16(1): 33–40.

Baerwald EF, d'Amours GH, Klug BJ, Barclay RM. 2008. Barotrauma is a significant cause of bat fatalities at wind turbines. Curr Biol 18(16): R695–96.

Balaban CD. 2002. Neural substrates linking balance control and anxiety. Physiol Behav 77: 469–75.

Balaban CD. 2004. Projections from the parabrachial nucleus to the vestibular nuclei: potential substrates for autonomic and limbic influences on vestibular responses. Brain Res 996: 126–37.

Balaban CD, Thayer JF. 2001. Neurological bases for balance-anxiety links. J Anxiety Disord 15: 53–79.

Balaban CD, Yates BJ. 2004. The vestibuloautonomic interactions: a teleologic perspective. Chapter 7 in *The Vestibular System*, ed. Highstein SM, Fay RR, Popper AN, pp. 286–342. Springer-Verlag, New York.

Baron, Robert Alex. 1970. *The Tyranny of Noise: The World's Most Prevalent Pollution, Who Causes It, How It's Hurting You, and How to Fight It*. St. Martin's Press, New York.

Beasley R, Clayton T, Crane J, von Mutius E, Lai CK, Montefort S, Stewart A; ISAAC Phase Three Study Group. 2008. Association between paracetamol use in infancy and childhood, and the risk of asthma, rhinoconjunctivitis, and eczema in children aged 6–7 years: analysis from Phase Three of the ISAAC programme. Lancet 372(9643): 1039–48.

Beranek LL. 2006. Basic acoustical quantities: levels and decibels. Chapter 1 in *Noise and Vibration Control and Engineering: Principles and Applications*, ed. Ver IL, Beranek LL, pp. 1–24. John Wiley & Sons, Hoboken, NJ.

Berglund B, Hassmen P, Job RFS. 1996. Sources and effects of low frequency noise. J Acoust Soc Am 99(5): 2985–3002.

Brandt T, Bartenstein P, Janek A, Dieterich M. 1998. Reciprocal inhibitory visual-vestibular interaction. Visual motion stimulation deactivates the parieto-insular vestibular cortex. Brain 121(Pt. 9): 1749–58.

Brandt T, Dieterich M. 1999. The vestibular cortex: its locations, functions, and disorders. Ann NY Acad Sci 871: 293–312.

Brandt T, Schautzer F, Hamilton DA, Bruning R, Markowitsch HJ, Kalla R, Darlington C, Smith P, Strupp M. 2005. Vestibular loss causes hippocampal atrophy and impaired spatial memory in humans. Brain 128: 2732–41.

Cappa S, Sterzi R, Vallar G, Bisiach E. 1987. Remission of hemineglect and anosognosia during vestibular stimulation. Neuropsychologia 25: 775–82.

Castelo Branco NAA. 1999. A unique case of vibroacoustic disease: a tribute to an extraordinary patient. Aviat Space Environ Med 70(3): A27–31.

Castelo Branco NAA, Aguas AP, Pereira AS, Monteiro E, Fragata JIG, Tavares F, Grande NR. 1999. The human pericardium in vibroacoustic disease. Aviat Space Environ Med 70(3): A54–62.

Castelo Branco NAA, Alves-Pereira M. 2004. Vibroacoustic disease. Noise Health 6(23): 3–20.

Castelo Branco NAA, Monteiro M, Ferreira JR, Monteiro E, Alves-Pereira M. 2007. Bronchoscopy in vibroacoustic disease III: electron microscopy. Inter-Noise 2007, August 28–31, Istanbul, Turkey.

Clark C, Martin R, van Kempen E, Alfred T, Head J, Davies HW, Haines MM, Barrio IL, Matheson M, Stansfeld SA. 2005. Exposure-effect relations between aircraft and road traffic noise exposure at school and reading comprehension: the RANCH project. Am J Epidemiol 163: 27–37.

Claussen CF, Claussen E. 1995. Neurootological contributions to the diagnostic follow-up after whiplash injuries. Acta Otolaryngol Suppl 520, Pt. 1: 53–56.

Coermann RR, Ziegenruecker GH, Wittwer AL, von Gierke HE. 1960. The passive dynamic mechanical properties of the human thorax-abdominal system and of the whole body system. Aerosp Med 31(6): 443–55.

Cohen S, Glass DC, Singer JE. 1973. Apartment noise, auditory discrimination, and reading ability in children. J Exp Soc Psychol 9: 407–22.

Colebatch JG, Day BL, Bronstein AM, Davies RA, Gresty MA, Luxon LM, Rothwell JC. 1998. Vestibular hypersensitivity to clicks is characteristic of the Tullio phenomenon. J Neurol Neurosurg Psychiatry 65: 670–78.

Colebatch JG, Halmagyi GM, Skuse NF. 1994. Myogenic potentials generated by a click-evoked vestibulocollic reflex. J Neurol Neurosurg Psychiatry 57(2): 190–97.

Curthoys IS, Kim J, McPhedran SK, Camp AJ. 2006. Bone conducted vibration selectively activates irregular primary otolithic vestibular neurons in the guinea pig. Exp Brain Res 175(2): 256–67.

Dieterich M, Brandt T. 2008. Functional brain imaging of peripheral and central vestibular disorders. Brain 131(10): 2538–52.

Eckhardt-Henn A, Breuer P, Thomalske C, Hoffmann SO, Hopf HC. 2003. Anxiety disorders and other psychiatric subgroups in patients complaining of dizziness. J Anxiety Disord 17(4): 369–88.

Edge PM, Mayes WH. 1966. Description of Langley low-frequency noise facility and study of human response to noise frequencies below 50 cps. NASA Technical Note, NASA TN D-3204, 11 pp.

Eriksson C, Rosenlund M, Pershagen G, Hilding A, Ostenson C-G, Bluhm G. 2007. Aircraft noise and incidence of hypertension. Epidemiology 18(6): 716–21.

Ernst A, Basta D, Seidl RO, Todt I, Scherer H, Clarke A. 2005. Management of posttraumatic vertigo. Otolaryngol Head Neck Surg 132(4): 554–58.

Evans GW, Maxwell L. 1997. Chronic noise exposure and reading deficits: the mediating effects of language acquisition. Environ Behav 29(5): 638–56.

Evans GW. 2006. Child development and the physical environment. Annu Rev Psychol 57: 423–51.

Fay RR, Simmons AM. 1999. The sense of hearing in fishes and amphibians. In *Comparative Hearing: Fish and Amphibians*, ed. Fay RR, Popper AN, pp. 269–317. Springer-Verlag, New York.

Feldmann J, Pitten FA. 2004. Effects of low-frequency noise on man: a case study. Noise Health 7(25): 23–28.

Findeis H, Peters E. 2004. Disturbing effects of low-frequency sound immissions and vibrations in residential buildings. Noise Health 6(23): 29–35.

Foudriat BA, Di Fabio RP, Anderson JH. 1993. Sensory organization of balance responses in children 3–6 years of age: a normative study with diagnostic implications. Int J Pediatr Otorhinolaryngol 27(3): 255–71.

Frey, Barbara J, and Hadden, Peter J. 2007. Noise radiation from wind turbines installed near homes: effects on health. 137 pp. www.windturbinenoisehealthhumanrights.com/wtnhhr_june2007.pdf.

Furman JM, Balaban CD, Jacob RG. 2001. Interface between vestibular dysfunction and anxiety: more than just psychogenicity. Otol Neurotol 22(3): 426–27.

Furman JM, Balaban CD, Jacob RG, Marcus DA. 2005. Migraine-anxiety related dizziness (MARD): a new disorder? J Neurol Neurosurg Psychiatry 76: 1–8.

Furman JM, Redfern MS, Jacob RG. 2006. Vestibulo-ocular function in anxiety disorders. J Vestib Res 16: 209–15.

Garcia J, Ervin FR. 1968. Gustatory-visceral and telereceptor-cutaneous conditioning: adaptation in internal and external milieus. Commun Behav Biol 1: 389–415.

Geminiani G, Bottini G. 1992. Mental representation and temporary recovery from unilateral neglect after vestibular stimulation. J Neurol Neurosurg Psychiatry 55(4): 332–33.

Giacomin J. 2005. Absorbed power of small children. Clin Biomech 20(4): 372–80.

Grimm RJ, Hemenway WG, Lebray PR, Black FO. 1989. The perilymph fistula syndrome defined in mild head trauma. Acta Otolaryngol Suppl 464: 1–40.

Gurney JG, van Wijngaarden E. 1999. Extremely low frequency electromagnetic fields (EMF) and brain cancer in adults and children: review and comment. Neuro Oncol 1(3): 212–20.

Hadamard J. 1996. *The Mathematician's Mind: The Psychology of Invention in the Mathematical Field.* Princeton University Press, Princeton, NJ.

Haines MM, Stansfeld SA, Job RFS, Berglund B, Head J. 2001. A follow-up study of effects of chronic aircraft noise exposure on child stress responses and cognition. Int J Epidemiol 30: 839–45.

Halberstadt A, Balaban CD. 2003. Organization of projections from the raphe nuclei to the vestibular nuclei in rats. Neuroscience 120(2): 573–94.

Hanes DA, McCollum G. 2006. Cognitive-vestibular interactions: a review of patient difficulties and possible mechanisms. J Vestib Res 16(3): 75–91.

Haralabidis AS, Dimakopoulou K, Vigna-Taglianti F, Giampaolo M, Borgini A, Dudley M-L, Pershagen G, Bluhm G, Houthuijs D, Babisch W, Velonakis M, Katsouyanni K, Jarup L. 2008. Acute effects of night-time noise exposure on blood pressure in populations living near airports. European Heart J 29(5): 658–64.

Harry, Amanda. 2007. Wind turbines, noise, and health. 32 pp. www.windturbinenoisehealthhumanrights.com/wtnoise_health_2007_a_barry.pdf.

Hedge, Alan. 2007. Department of Design and Environmental Analysis, Cornell University. Syllabus/lecture notes for DEA 350:

Whole-body vibration (January), found at http://ergo.human.cornell.edu/studentdownloads/DEA325pdfs/Human%20Vibration.pdf.

Hillis HE, Caramazza A. 1995. Spatially specific deficits in processing graphemic representations in reading and writing. Brain Lang 48(3): 263–308.

Hygge S, Evans GW, Bullinger M. 2002. A prospective study of some effects of aircraft noise on cognitive performance in schoolchildren. Psychol Sci 13: 469–74.

Indovina I, Maffei V, Bosco G, Zago M, Macaluso E, Lacquaniti F. 2005. Representation of visual gravitational motion in the human vestibular cortex. Science 308: 416–19.

Ishizaki K, Mori N, Takeshima T, Fukuhara Y, Ijiri T, Kusumi M, Yasui K, Kowa H, Nakashima K. 2002. Static stabilometry in patients with migraine and tension-type headache during a headache-free period. Psychiatry Clin Neurosci 56(1): 85–90.

Ising H, Braun C. 2000. Acute and chronic endocrine effects of noise: review of the research conducted at the Institute for Water, Soil and Air Hygiene. Noise Health 7: 7–24.

Ising H, Ising M. 2002. Chronic cortisol increases in the first half of the night caused by road traffic noise. Noise Health 4: 13–21.

Jacob RG, Furman JM, Durrant JD, Turner SM. 1996. Panic, agoraphobia, and vestibular dysfunction. Am J Psychiatry 153(4): 503–12.

Jacob RG, Redfern MS, Furman JM. 2009. Space and motion discomfort and abnormal balance control in patients with anxiety disorders. J Neurol Neurosurg Psychiatry 80(1): 74–78. E-pub 2008 July 24.

Jacob RG, Woody SR, Clark DB, Lilienfeld SO, Hirsch BE, Kucera GD, Furman JM, Durrant JD. 1993. Discomfort with space and motion: a possible marker of vestibular dysfunction assessed by the

Situational Characteristics Questionnaire. J Psychopathol Behav Assess 15(4): 299–324.

Jarup L, Babisch W, Houthuijs D, Pershagen G, Katsouyanni K, Cadum E, Dudley M-L, Savigny P, Seiffert I, Swart W, Breugelmans O, Bluhm G, Selander J, Haralabidis A, Dimakopoulou K, Sourtzi P, Velonakis M, Vigna-Taglianti F. 2008. Hypertension and exposure to noise near airports: the HYENA study. Environ Health Perspect 116(3): 329–33.

Johansen C. 2004. Electromagnetic fields and health effects: epidemiologic studies of cancer, diseases of the central nervous system and arrhythmia-related heart disease. Scand J Work Environ Health 30 Suppl 1: 1–30.

Kamperman GW, James RR. 2008a. Simple guidelines for siting wind turbines to prevent health risks. Noise-Con, July 28–31, Institute of Noise Control Engineering/USA.

Kamperman GW, James RR. 2008b. The "how to" guide to siting wind turbines to prevent health risks from sound. 44 pp. www.windturbinesyndrome.com.

Karlsen HE, Piddington RW, Enger PS, Sand O. 2004. Infrasound initiates directional fast-start escape responses in juvenile roach *Rutilus rutilus*. J Exp Biol 207(Pt. 24): 4185–93.

Kayan A, Hood JD. 1984. Neuro-otological manifestations of migraine. Brain 107:1123–42.

Lee H, Sohn SI, Jung DK, Cho YW, Lim JG, Yi SD, Yi HA. 2002. Migraine and isolated recurrent vertigo of unknown cause. Neurol Res 24(7): 663–65.

Lercher P, Evans GW, Meis M. 2003. Ambient noise and cognitive processes among primary schoolchildren. Environ Behav 35(6): 725–35.

Leventhall, Geoff. 2004. Notes on low frequency noise from wind turbines with special reference to the Genesis Power Ltd. Proposal near Waiuku, NZ. Prepared for Genesis Power/Hegley Acoustic Consultants, June 4.

Lipton RB, Bigal ME, Diamond M, Freitag F, Reed ML, Stewart WF; AMPP Advisory Group. 2007. Migraine prevalence, disease burden, and the need for preventive therapy. Neurology 68(5): 343–49.

Maguire EA, Valentine ER, Wilding JM, Kapur N. 2003. Routes to remembering: the brains behind superior memory. Nat Neurosci 6(1): 90–95.

Marcus DA, Furman JM, Balaban CD. 2005. Motion sickness in migraine sufferers. Expert Opin Pharmacother 6(15): 2691–97.

Martinho Pimenta AJ, Castelo Branco NAA. 1999. Neurological aspects of vibroacoustic disease. Aviat Space Environ Med 70(3): A91–95.

Mast FW, Merfeld DM, Kosslyn SM. 2006. Visual mental imagery during caloric vestibular stimulation. Neuropsychologia 44(1): 101–9.

Minor, LB. 2003. Labyrinthine fistulae: pathobiology and management. Curr Opin Otolaryngol Head Neck Surg 11(5): 340–46.

Mittelstaedt H. 1996. Somatic graviception. Biol Psychol 42(1–2): 53–74.

Mittelstaedt H. 1999. The role of the otoliths in perception of the vertical and in path integration. Ann NY Acad Sci 871: 334–44.

Monteiro M, Ferreira JR, Alves-Pereira M, Castelo Branco NAA. 2007. Bronchoscopy in vibroacoustic disease I: "pink lesions." Inter-Noise 2007, August 28–31, Istanbul, Turkey.

Murakami DM, Erkman L, Hermanson O, Rosenfeld MG, Fuller CA. 2002. Evidence for vestibular regulation of autonomic functions in a mouse genetic model. Proc Natl Acad Sci USA 99(26): 17078–82.

Muzet A, Miedema H. 2005. Short-term effects of transportation noise on sleep with specific attention to mechanisms and possible health impact. Draft paper presented at the Third Meeting on Night Noise Guidelines, WHO European Center for Environment and Health, Lisbon, Portugal, April 26–28. Pp. 5–7 in *Report on the Third Meeting on Night Noise Guidelines*, available at www.euro.who.int/Document/NOH/3rd_NNG_final_rep_rev.pdf.

National Institute on Deafness and Other Communication Disorders, USA, website, "Prevalence of chronic tinnitus." 2009. www.nidcd.nih.gov/health/statistics/prevalence.htm.

National Research Council. 2007. *Environmental Impacts of Wind-Energy Projects*. The National Academies Press, Washington, DC. 185 pp.

Neuhauser H, Leopold M, von Brevern M, Arnold G, Lempert T. 2001. The interactions of migraine, vertigo, and migrainous vertigo. Neurology 56: 436–41.

Oliveira MJR, Pereira AS, Castelo Branco NAA, Grande NR, Aguas AP. 2002. In utero and postnatal exposure of Wistar rats to low frequency/high intensity noise depletes the tracheal epithelium of ciliated cells. Lung 179: 225–32.

Oliveira MJR, Pereira AS, Ferreira PG, Guinaraes L, Freitas D, Carvalho APO, Grande NR, Aguas AP. 2004. Arrest in ciliated cell expansion on the bronchial lining of adult rats caused by chronic exposure to industrial noise. Environ Res 97: 282–86.

Omalu BI, DeKosky ST, Minster RL, Kamboh MI, Hamilton RL, Wecht CH. 2005. Chronic traumatic encephalopathy in a National Football League player. Neurosurgery 57: 128–34.

Omalu BI, DeKosky ST, Hamilton RL, Minster RL, Kamboh MI, Shakir AM, Wecht CH. 2006. Chronic traumatic encephalopathy in a National Football League player: part II. Neurosurgery 59: 1086–93.

Pawlaczyk-Luszczynska M, Dudarewicz A, Waszkowska M, Szymczak W, Sliwinska-Kowalska M. 2005. The impact of low-frequency noise on human mental performance. Int J Occup Med Environ Health 18(2): 185–98.

Pedersen E. 2007. Human response to wind turbine noise: perception, annoyance and moderating factors. PhD diss., Occupational and Environmental Medicine, Department of Public Health and Community Medicine, Göteborg University, Göteborg, Sweden. 86 pp.

Pedersen E, Bouma J, Bakker R, van den Berg GP. 2008. Response to wind turbine noise in the Netherlands. J Acoust Soc Am 123(5): 3536 (abstract).

Pedersen E, Persson Waye K. 2004. Perception and annoyance due to wind turbine noise: a dose-response relationship. J Acoust Soc Am 116(6): 3460–70.

Pedersen E, Persson Waye K. 2007. Wind turbine noise, annoyance and self-reported health and wellbeing in different living environments. Occup Environ Med 64(7): 480–86.

Pereira AS, Grande NR, Monteiro E, Castelo Branco MSN, Castelo Branco NAA. 1999. Morphofunctional study of rat pleural mesothelial cells exposed to low frequency noise. Aviat Space Environ Med 70(3): A78–85.

Perna G, Dario A, Caldirola D, Stefania B, Cesarani A, Bellodi L. 2001. Panic disorder: the role of the balance system. J Psychiatr Res 35(5): 279–86.

Persson Waye K. 2004. Effects of low frequency noise on sleep. Noise Health 6(23): 87–91.

Phipps, Robyn. 2007. Evidence of Dr. Robyn Phipps in the matter of Moturimu wind farm application heard before the Joint Commissioners, March 8–26. Palmerston North, New Zealand. 43 pp. www.wind-watch.org/documents/wp-content/uploads/phipps-moturimutestimony.pdf.

Rasmussen G. 1982. Human body vibration exposure and its measurement. Bruel & Kjaer Technical Paper No. 1, Naerum, Denmark. Abstract: Rasmussen G. 1983. Human body vibration exposure and its measurement. J Acoust Soc Am 73(6): 2229.

Redfern MS, Furman JM, Jacob RG. 2007. Visually induced postural sway in anxiety disorders. J Anxiety Disord 21(5): 704–16. NIH Public Access Author Manuscript, pp. 1–14.

Redfern MS, Yardley L, Bronstein AM. 2001. Visual influences on balance. J Anxiety Disord 15(1–2): 81–94.

Reid A, Cottingham CA, Marchbanks RJ. 1993. The prevalence of perilymphatic hypertension in subjects with tinnitus: a pilot study. Scand Audiol 22: 61–63.

Rennie, Gary. 2009. Wind farm noise limits urged. *The Windsor Star* (Ontario, Canada). February 24.

Rilke, Rainer Maria. 1981. "The Neighbor." *Selected Poems of Rainer Maria Rilke: A Translation from the German and Commentary by Robert Bly*, p. 93. Harper & Row, New York.

Rilke, Rainer Maria. 1991. "The Angels," trans. Snow. *The Book of Images: A Bilingual Edition*, rev. ed., p. 31. North Point Press, New York.

Rinne T, Bronstein AM, Rudge P, Gresty MA, Luxon LM. 1998. Bilateral loss of vestibular function: clinical findings in 53 patients. J Neurol 245(6–7): 314–21.

Rosenhall U, Johansson G, Orndahl G. 1996. Otoneurologic and audiologic findings in fibromyalgia. Scand J Rehabil Med 28(4): 225–32.

Salt AN. 2004. Acute endolymphatic hydrops generated by exposure of the ear to nontraumatic low-frequency tones. J Assoc Res Otolaryngol 5(2): 203–14.

Sand O, Karlsen HE. 1986. Detection of infrasound by the Atlantic cod. J Exp Biol. 125: 197–204.

Sand O, Karlsen HE. 2000. Detection of infrasound and linear acceleration in fishes. Phil Trans R Soc Lond B 355: 1295–98.

Sand O, Karlsen HE, Knudsen FR. 2008. Comment on "Silent research vessels are not quiet" [J Acoust Soc Am 2007; 121(4): EL145–50]. J Acoust Soc Am 123(4): 1831–33.

Saunders RD, Jefferys JGR. 2002. Weak electric field interactions in the central nervous system. Health Physics 83(3): 366–75.

Schlindwein P, Mueller M, Bauermann T, Brandt T, Stoeter P, Dieterich M. 2008. Cortical representation of saccular vestibular stimulation: VEMPs in fMRI. Neuroimage 39: 19–31.

Schore, Allan N. 1994. *Affect Regulation and the Origin of the Self: The Neurobiology of Emotional Development*. Lawrence Earlbaum Associates, Hillsdale, NJ. 700 pp.

Sinclair, Upton. 1935. *I, Candidate for Governor: And How I Got Licked*. Farrar & Rinehart, New York.

Sokal RR, Rohlf FJ. 1969. *Biometry*. W. H. Freeman, San Francisco.

Staud R, Cannon RC, Mauderli AP, Robinson ME, Price DD, Vierck CJ Jr. 2003. Temporal summation of pain from mechanical stimulation of muscle tissue in normal controls and subjects with fibromyalgia syndrome. Pain 102: 87–95.

Steindl R, Kunz K, Schrott-Fischer A, Scholtz AW. 2006. Effect of age and sex on maturation of sensory systems and balance control. Dev Med Child Neurol 48(6): 477–82.

Stewart WF, Simon D, Shechter A, Lipton RB. 1995. Population variation in migraine prevalence: a meta-analysis. J Clin Epidemiol 48(2): 269–80.

Styles P, Stimpson I, Toon S, England R, and Wright M. 2005. Microseismic and infrasound monitoring of low frequency noise and vibrations from wind farms: recommendations on the siting of wind farms in the vicinity of Eskdalemuir, Scotland. 125 pp. www.esci.keele.ac.uk/geophysics/News/windfarm_monitoring.html.

Takahashi Y, Kanada K, Yonekawa Y, Harada N. 2005. A study on the relationship between subjective unpleasantness and body surface vibrations induced by high-level low-frequency pure tones. Ind Health 43: 580–87.

Takahashi Y, Yonekawa Y, Kanada K, Maeda S. 1999. A pilot study on the human body vibration induced by low-frequency noise. Ind Health 37: 28–35.

Todd NPMc, Rosengren SM, Colebatch JG. 2008. Tuning and sensitivity of the human vestibular system to low-frequency vibration. Neurosci Lett 444: 36–41.

Todd NP, Rosengren SM, Colebatch JG. 2009. A utricular origin of frequency tuning to low-frequency vibration in the human vestibular system? Neurosci Lett 451(3): 175–80.

Uzun-Coruhlu H, Curthoys IS, Jones AS. 2007. Attachment of utricular and saccular maculae to the temporal bone. Hear Res 233(1–2): 77–85.

Vaitl D, Mittelstaedt H, Baisch F. 2002. Shifts in blood volume alter the perception of posture: further evidence for somatic graviception. Int J Psychophysiol 44(1): 1–11.

van den Berg, GP. 2004a. Do wind turbines produce significant low frequency sound levels? 11th International Meeting on Low Frequency Noise and Vibration and Its Control, Maastricht, Netherlands, August 30-September 1.

van den Berg, GP. 2004b. Effects of the wind profile at night on wind turbine sound. J Sound Vib 277: 955–70.

van den Berg, GP. 2005. The beat is getting stronger: the effect of atmospheric stability on low frequency modulated sound of wind turbines. J Low Freq Noise Vib Active Contr 24(1): 1–24.

van den Berg, GP. 2006. The sound of high winds: the effect of atmospheric stability on wind turbine sound and microphone noise. PhD diss., University of Groningen, Netherlands. 177 pp. http://irs.ub.rug.nl/ppn/294294104.

van den Berg GP, Pedersen E, Bakker R, Bouma J. 2008a. Wind farm aural and visual impact in the Netherlands. J Acoust Soc Am 123(5): 3682 (abstract).

van den Berg GP, Pedersen E, Bouma J, Bakker R. 2008b. Project WINDFARMperception: visual and acoustic impact of wind turbine farms on residents. Final report, June 3. 63 pp. Summary: http://umcg.wewi.eldoc.ub.rug.nl/FILES/root/Rapporten/2008/WINDFARMperception/WFp-final-summary.pdf. Entire report: https://dspace.hh.se/dspace/bitstream/2082/2176/1/WFp-final.pdf.

von Gierke HE. 1971. Biodynamic models and their applications. J Acoust Soc Am 50(6): 1397–413.

von Gierke HE, Parker DE. 1994. Differences in otolith and abdominal viscera graviceptor dynamics: implications for motion sickness and perceived body position. Aviat Space Environ Med 65(8): 747–51.

Vuilleumier P, Ortigue S, Brugger P. 2004. The number space and neglect. Cortex 40(2): 399–410.

Welgampola MS, Rosengren SM, Halmagyi GM, Colebatch JG. 2003. Vestibular activation by bone conducted sound. J Neurol Neurosurg Psychiatry 74: 711–18.

Welgampola MS, Day BL. 2006. Craniocentric body-sway responses to 500 Hz bone-conducted tones in man. J Physiol 577(1): 81–95.

Wilson TD, Cotter LA, Draper JA, Misra SP, Rice CD, Cass SP, Yates BJ. 2006. Vestibular inputs elicit patterned changes in limb blood flow in conscious cats. J Physiol 575(2): 671–84.

World Health Organization. 1999. *Guidelines for Community Noise*, ed. Berglund B, Lindvall T, Schwela DH. 159 pp. www.who.int/docstore/peh/noise/guidelines2.html.

Yardley L, Britton J, Lear S, Bird J, Luxon LM. 1995. Relationship between balance system function and agoraphobic avoidance. Behav Res Ther 33(4): 435–39.

Yardley L, Luxon LM, Lear S, Britton J, Bird J. 1994. Vestibular and posturographic test results in people with symptoms of panic and agoraphobia. J Audiol Med 3: 58–65.

Yates BJ, Aoki M, Burchill P, Bronstein AM. 1999. Cardiovascular responses elicited by linear acceleration in humans. Exp Brain Res 125: 476–84.

Zorzi M, Priftis K, Umilta C. 2002. Brain damage: neglect disrupts the mental number line. Nature 417: 138–39.

Referee reports

Dr. Pierpont's report deserves publication. Although the case numbers are not large, the careful documentation of serious physical, neurological, and emotional problems provoked by living close to wind turbines must be brought to the attention of physicians who, like me, were unaware of them until now.

By a well devised questionnaire/interview the author has been able to obtain data demonstrating the correlation of symptoms induced by active wind turbines, the improvement/resolution of symptoms when the interviewees have moved away, and the re-emergence of the same symptoms when returning to their homes near the turbines.

With the pressure on our governments to go "green," eliminating coal-powered sources of electricity, the United States Environmental Protection Agency in conjunction with Dr. Pierpont and this report should expand this investigation and establish the necessary guidelines for creating wind turbine "farms" and protect those near to them.

> JEROME S. HALLER, MD, Professor of Neurology and Pediatrics (retired 2008), Albany Medical College, Albany, New York. Dr. Haller is a member of the American Academy of Pediatrics, the American Academy of Neurology (Child Neurology Section), and the Child Neurology Society.

June 10, 2008

Dr. Pierpont's study addresses an under-reported facet of Noise Induced Illnesses in a fashion that is detailed in its historical documentation, multi-systemic in its approach and descriptions, and painstakingly and informatively referenced.

The study provides a scientific underpinning for viewing symptom complexes that are generally unappreciated and difficult to comprehend for the great majority of medical practitioners who have to rely, in their daily practice, on identifying anatomical or chemical abnormalities in order to establish a diagnosis. This approach opens up an avenue to diagnosis and comprehension that was exciting to me, and, I feel, would excite the interest of a large group of practitioners who are open to looking at the patient as a person, rather than as a machine. It will encourage physicians to listen carefully to their patients and place their patients in the environment rather than the lab.

Dr. Pierpont's study is particularly important because of the present energy crisis (and the role of environment-changing technologies to address it), it is very readable, extremely well referenced and most informative. The patients described are true "sufferers" (the root of the word patient) whose lives have been seriously disrupted. As I mentioned above, it is particularly relevant at a time when wind energy technology and its applications are growing worldwide. It alerts the medical profession to the potential for illness caused by low frequency vibrations. It encourages the medical profession to scrutinize other, new energy technology for potential side effects.

It is my hope that this study, when published, will stimulate research not only on the deleterious effects of low frequency vibration on the human species, but also on its effects upon the animal world in general. I would also hope that the symptom complexes that are described will be studied more intensely so as to gain a greater understanding of the human body as regards its physiology and pathophysiology. I am convinced that successful analysis of the physical forces that impact on humans will add an important dimension to our understanding of physiology and disease states. This study opens up the area of low frequency vibration to the medical community. Other physical forces, both mechanical and electrical, could play a role in certain human diseases. This study could encourage recognition of the research accomplishments in analyzing disease states through analysis of these physical forces.

Since the analysis of these forces is presently outside of the medical model of disease diagnosis, many of these sufferers have been labeled as having a purely psychological problem. The author has provided a basis to describe such a group of symptom complexes as pathophysiological, and I applaud her.

> JOEL F. LEHRER, MD, Fellow of the American College of Surgeons, Clinical Professor of Otolaryngology, University of Medicine & Dentistry of New Jersey. Formerly Professor of Otolaryngology, Mount Sinai School of Medicine, New York, New York.

June 29, 2008

I congratulate you on your case-series investigation on Wind Turbine Syndrome. That is, the conception, the data gathering, the analysis and the write-up. As an epidemiologist I fully appreciate your truly remarkable effort, one that smacks of being well done and with a full respect for honest inquiry. Given your initial suspicions on this matter, your high level of scientific integrity is revealed both in your design decisions and in your writing, both of which are of the highest order.

What you have accomplished is, at once, both remarkable and limited (as you fully appreciate). I see several noteworthy outcomes of your admirable and remarkable presentation of this case-series report on Wind Turbine Syndrome from your perspective as a concerned, practicing physician from the community.

1) Creation of a case-definition for Wind Turbine Syndrome. You have initiated a critical first step needed to convert "an issue of concern" into a "researchable topic" by your putting forth a clear case-definition of Wind Turbine Syndrome, including the recognition and development of a newly defined symptom which you document and call Visceral Vibratory Vestibular Disturbance (VVVD).

2) Creation of a thoughtful list of future research suggestions into Wind Turbine Syndrome. By your deep and obvious commitment to get at the truth of this matter, you have proposed a thoughtful and rich list of directions for others to pursue in this line of inquiry, something that involved investigators can uniquely do as a result of the depth of their intellectual investment in the line of inquiry.

3) Candidly presented an insightful list of the limitations of your case-series study. It instills confidence in the reader that you, indeed, conducted a study aimed at discovering the truth of the matter, which always demands candor and insights from the investigator who best knows the range of limitations, from minor up to major (if any), in one's own study.

As you fully appreciate, the biggest overall limitation of your work is the lack of "generalizability" of the specific findings to broader populations due to the specific (but both appropriate and necessary) eligibility criteria for subjects in your case-series. This is nothing to worry about, merely something to appreciate and build upon, as this limitation is inherent to any early-stage epidemiologic investigation into an evolving subject area.

You have laid a remarkable, high quality, and honest foundation for others to build upon with the next stages of scientific investigation. In doing so, you have made a commendable, thorough, careful, honest, and significant contribution to the study of (what we can now call) Wind Turbine Syndrome.

> RALPH V. KATZ, DMD, MPH, PhD, Fellow of the American College of Epidemiology, Professor and Chair, Department of Epidemiology & Health Promotion, New York University College of Dentistry, New York, New York

October 5, 2008

Dr. Pierpont has gathered a strong series of case studies of deleterious effects on the health and well being of many people living near large wind turbines. Furthermore she has reviewed medical studies that support a plausible physiological mechanism directly linking low frequency noise and vibration, like that produced by wind turbines, which may not in itself be reported as irritating, to potentially debilitating effects on the inner ear and other sensory systems associated with balance and sense of position. Thus the effects are likely to have a physiological component, rather than being exclusively psychological.

More extensive and statistically controlled observations may be needed to discover just how far from the turbines the deleterious effects occur, and in what proportion of the population. However, it is already clear that many people are affected at far greater distances than the minimum set-backs currently allowed between turbines and residences. Accordingly, it would be prudent to establish much longer set-backs from houses as a criterion for siting new turbines, pending further studies on this newly documented "wind turbine syndrome." Documentation of the syndrome itself is strong evidence that current set-backs are woefully inadequate.

HENRY S. HORN, PhD, Professor of Ecology and Evolutionary Biology, and Associate of the Princeton Environmental Institute, Princeton University, Princeton, New Jersey

October 17, 2008

About the author

I am a New Englander by many generations, growing up in a family of teachers and writers. My grandfather, like me, was a physician and ecologist. After being blessed by a fine elementary school (New Canaan Country School, 1970) and high school (Milton Academy, 1973), I attended Yale on a National Merit Scholarship, graduating in 1977 with a BA in biology. I earned a PhD (1985) in behavioral ecology at Princeton (training that I use substantially in my work in behavioral pediatrics), did a post-doctoral fellowship in ornithology at the American Museum of Natural History (NYC), and, as an over-the-hill woman of thirty-two, went to the Johns Hopkins University School of Medicine, where I earned the MD degree (1991).

I wanted to give my ecology training a human face. I chose the face of a child, becoming a pediatrician by completing internship at the Children's National Medical Center, Washington, DC, and residency at the Dartmouth-Hitchcock Medical Center, Lebanon, NH (because my husband, a country lad, detested Washington).

Despite his feelings toward Washington, and his improbable name (Calvin Luther Martin), my husband is a respectable man (retired Rutgers University professor and author of well-known scholarly books). Our two children (my stepchildren) are grown and have made us grandparents.

I am 54 years old.

I am an unabashed lover of wildness. I did my PhD research living in a tent in the Amazon jungle for several years, studying bird behavior. In pursuit of wildness and native cultures, my husband and I lived for another several years with Yup'ik Eskimos on the

Alaska tundra, near the Bering Sea, where I became chief of pediatrics at a native-run hospital. Likewise, we spent a summer living on the Navajo reservation, as I did a sub-internship in medical school.

For three years I ran a general pediatrics practice in Malone, Franklin County, NY (poorest county in the state), where I was, as well, the pediatrician for the St. Regis Mohawk Nation (Hogansburg, NY). For the next three years (2000–03) I was Senior Attending in Pediatrics at Bassett Healthcare, Cooperstown, NY (and, must confess, never darkened the door of the Baseball Hall of Fame). Bassett is a teaching hospital of Columbia University, and I was Assistant Clinical Professor of Pediatrics at Columbia's College of Physicians & Surgeons.

I am a board-certified pediatrician licensed in the State of New York and Fellow of the American Academy of Pediatrics. These days I limit my practice to behavioral medicine, seeing both adults and (chiefly) children, drawing my patients from an extensive area of rural upstate New York. I have had considerable post-graduate training in behavioral medicine, which I have been able to integrate with my doctoral training in behavioral ecology.

My research on Wind Turbine Syndrome is the offspring of behavioral medicine married to behavioral ecology.

Most of all, I love what I do. I believe in compassion and grace and get tremendous pleasure and joy out of my patients. (To children's delight, I carefully count their toes.) I run my practice out of my home as an old-fashioned doctor's office. Cheerful, light, airy, perhaps the faint smell of my husband's burnt toast wafting through the house. Norman Rockwell's America.